THE
Vitamin Alphabet

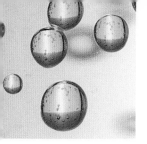

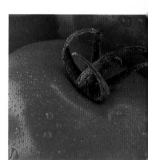

THE
Vitamin Alphabet

Your guide to vitamins, minerals and food supplements

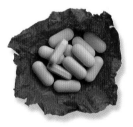

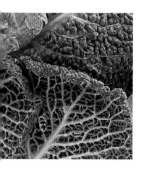

Dr Christina Scott-Moncrieff MB ChB MFHOM

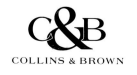

COLLINS & BROWN

First published in Great Britain in 1999
by Collins & Brown Limited
London House
Great Eastern Wharf
Parkgate Road
London SW11 4NQ

Distributed in the United States and Canada by Sterling Publishing Co,
387 Park Avenue South, New York, NY 10016 USA

British Library Cataloguing-in-Publication Data:
A catalogue record for this book
is available from the British Library.

ISBN 1 85585 681 6

Designer: Becky Willis, The Bridgewater Book Company
Special photography: Ian Parsons

Reproduction by Hong Kong Graphic & Printing Ltd
Printed and bound in Hong Kong by Dai Nippon

Contents

How to use this book

In developed countries today, the supermarkets and food shops are filled with a wider choice of food than has ever previously been available, even to the affluent. Despite this, successive scientific papers have shown that substantial numbers of people living in these countries do not obtain enough vitamins and minerals, even though their diets do not lack calories.

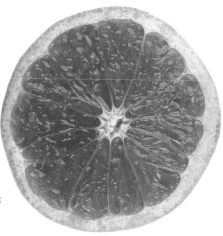

Food: the great healer

In the 1970s, researchers began to ask why people living in less affluent countries appeared to be less likely to develop cancer and heart disease, and often lived longer than people in Western countries, who had much greater access to medical services. The answer lay in the fact that the diets of people in these poorer countries are usually rich in fruit, vegetables and whole-grain cereals. The researchers found that these unprocessed foods apparently contained substances that conferred some protection against various diseases, and they were also rich in minerals and vitamins.

A well-balanced nutritionally rich diet is the foundation of good health, and such a diet should provide all the vitamins and minerals that are needed. Some healthy people eating a good, balanced diet take vitamin and mineral supplements to make sure that their daily requirements are met. There is no harm in this.

There are times, however, when the body does need more vitamins and minerals than can easily be obtained from the diet. Taking supplements can thus be worth considering during periods of growth, especially adolescence, illness and stress, or when the diet is inadequate as a result of loss of appetite, during a weight-loss programme, or when there is exposure to pollution. Women will also have greater needs during pregnancy and when breast feeding (see p110–111).

One thing that must be stressed, however, is that despite their potential benefits, vitamin and mineral supplements cannot replace a good diet. In addition to minerals and vitamins, a healthy diet contains protein, fat and carbohydrate, and a wide variety of other chemical compounds, many of which are only just being identified. All these components have their own specific health-giving functions.

How much is enough?

For many years, doctors, scientists and governments have been trying to determine the amounts of minerals and vitamins that are needed in the human diet. Originally, it was thought that the absence of the diseases caused by severe deficiencies of minerals and vitamins indicated that the intake was adequate.

This is too simplistic, and it is now recognized that minor deficiencies can give rise to symptoms without causing disease. For example, a lack of B-vitamins can result in insomnia, irritability and sugar cravings, and these are symptoms that most people would prefer to be without, even though they do not constitute an illness with a formal diagnosis.

As yet there is no world agreement on what constitutes an adequate intake of minerals and vitamins. However, various governments have now published tables recommending the amounts that are believed to supply the needs of most healthy people. But these do not take into account the extra needs of differing lifestyles (see introduction to chapter 5, p130–131).

What are vitamins and what do they do?

Vitamins are chemical compounds that occur in foods and have been shown to be essential for life. Many of them can also be produced, at least in limited amounts, in the body. However, the food we eat is our main source of vitamins and over the millennia the human body has adapted to obtaining vitamins from a range of whole, natural foods with maximum efficiency.

Vitamins are needed only in small amounts to be effective, but they are essential for the basic functions of the body. These include the release of energy stored in food, the formation and repair of tissues, reproduction, digestion, the production of urine and sweat, the secretion of hormones and the ability to resist disease and infection. An insufficient intake of vitamins can result in poor general health or, if the deficiency is severe, specific illnesses.

What are minerals and what do they do?

Minerals are chemical elements that are key components of our bodies, including teeth, bones, blood cells, and soft tissues. They are essential for the normal activity of muscles and the balance of fluid in the circulation and the tissues, and within the cells of the body.

Minerals, unlike many vitamins, cannot be made in the body, and have to be obtained from food. Their availability in the food we eat depends to some extent on the natural mineral deposits found in the land on which the food is produced.

We know from the sales of vitamins, that many people are aware of

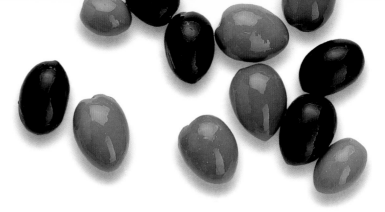

the possibility of vitamin deficiencies, but mineral deficiencies may be more common in the Western world. This is partly because intensive farming has resulted in the loss of some minerals from the soil. These are not routinely replaced where chemical fertilizers are being used instead of more traditional agricultural methods. In addition, many people opt for highly processed foods, such as white flours, rice and sugar, from which substantial amounts of the minerals that were originally contained in the whole plant have been removed.

Herbal helpers

Herbs are plants with medicinal and aromatic qualities. Their healing properties have long been harnessed by human beings to maintain or restore health. Some of the beneficial properties of herbs have been discovered by chance. This herbal help is partly pharmacological and partly because many herbs are themselves rich sources of minerals and vitamins. Guidance for the safe use of herbal supplements is given on page 92.

Using this book

This book is not designed to be read from cover to cover, but to be used for reference by you and your family.

CHAPTERS 1 and 2 provide an introduction to vitamins and minerals. They explain what these nutrients do, which foods contain them, how to check for deficiencies, and when you might need extra amounts.

CHAPTER 3 introduces a selection of herbs, both culinary and medicinal, that may be useful as extra aids to your health and fitness.

CHAPTER 4 is a guide to your individual needs from infancy to old age. The advice and recommendations given can be studied in detail in the first three chapters.

CHAPTER 5 contains the officially recommended daily intakes of minerals and vitamins.

If you think you need to take vitamin and mineral supplements

• Check with your doctor or pharmacist that it is safe to start a supplement if you are already taking other medication, or have any long-term medical condition

• Do not exceed the manufacturer's recommended dose without professional advice

• Remember that some minerals and vitamins can be toxic in excess amounts, so if you are taking one as part of more than one supplement you should check with your doctor or pharmacist that your total dose is safe

• Stop taking the supplement if you experience any side effects

• Always seek professional advice for a correct diagnosis about any symptoms you experience

A guide to vitamin and mineral supplements

Vitamin and mineral supplements are prepared in several ways:

NATURAL VITAMIN SUPPLEMENTS are derived from food sources and usually contain a natural mix of vitamins and other derivatives from the original source. Common sources are yeast, liver, maize (corn), soy, rosehips and alfalfa. Any allergic reaction may be to the extra ingredients rather than to the vitamin itself. In general the doses are not very high.

SYNTHETIC VITAMIN SUPPLEMENTS are made in a laboratory and contain the exact chemical formula of the vitamin. Doses are usually higher than the natural supplements, and some preparations contain vitamins from both sources.

CHELATED MINERALS have been specially prepared by the manufacturers to facilitate the absorption of the mineral in the body.

ORGANIC and NON-ORGANIC are terms that are not usually used in the agricultural sense (i.e. organic being produced without chemical additives). A chemist regards all vitamins as organic because they all contain carbon atoms. Minerals are not organic, because they are chemical elements, but some of them (notably selenium and chromium) are more easily absorbed if they are attached to carbon during manufacture.

VITAMINS and MINERALS can be presented in various forms:

TABLETS have a long shelf life. They contain additives known as fillers, packers and stabilizers that can cause allergic reactions.

CAPSULES are used for fat-soluble vitamins and powdered formulations. They are usually made of animal gelatine. When buying oil or oil capsules, it is important to check that the oil has been 'cold pressed' during preparation to avoid adverse chemical changes.

POWDERED PREPARATIONS are the most rapidly absorbed formulations, but are often the least palatable. They are usually free of additives.

LIQUIDS can contain colouring agents and sweeteners (as can children's chewable formulations).

Getting to know your vitamins

Over the years the official list of vitamins has grown longer, and will probably continue to do so as the various natural chemical compounds that occur in food are isolated and studied. Compared with the amount of food that we eat, vitamins are needed only in very small amounts, and they do not of themselves supply any energy or contribute to the tissues of the body. However, they facilitate the various biochemical processes of the body and are often known as micronutrients.

As our knowledge grows, a number of substances once considered to be vitamins are no longer believed to be essential to life, and so are no longer recognized formally as vitamins. Because they are nevertheless still widely known, we have listed and defined them in this chapter.

By convention, vitamins are usually divided into two groups: those that dissolve in water and those that dissolve in fat. However, a convenient way to take vitamin supplements is to choose a multi-vitamin formulation that contains both groups.

The water-soluble vitamins include the B-vitamins and vitamins C and P. With the exception of vitamin B12, these vitamins are mainly found in foods that are derived from plants and are eliminated quickly from the body in the urine and sweat. Foods and supplements that contain these water-soluble vitamins are most effective when taken several times a day. Vitamin B12, however, comes from animal foods and enough to last for several years can be stored in the liver.

In nature, many of the B-vitamins occur in the same foods, and they work together in the body. If supplements are taken to 'top up' the diet it is best to take the B-vitamins together in a balanced formulation. Individual B-vitamins, taken for specific purposes can then be added for short periods, but if you wish to take them long-term it is important to avoid imbalances (see individual B-vitamins in this chapter). Vitamins C and P also occur together in nature and supplements should, preferably, contain both.

The fat-soluble vitamins, A, D, E, F and K, are present in foods derived from both plants and animals. They are stored in the body, so foods and supplements that contain them do not need to be eaten as frequently as those containing water-soluble vitamins. Indeed, toxicity may become a problem if fat soluble vitamins are regularly taken in excess, and this is a particular concern with vitamins A and D. If you take more than one supplement containing these two vitamins, it is important to check with a doctor or pharmacist that you are not taking too much.

Vitamin B1
thiamine

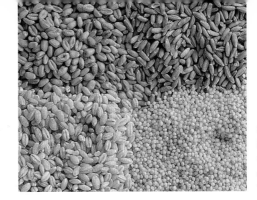

LEFT *The germ and bran of wheat, rice and other grains are rich sources of vitamin B1.*

Vitamin B1 is needed for energy production, particularly in the muscles, including those of the heart. By maintaining the health of the nervous system, it helps to combat disorders of the nerves, such as neuritis, and psychological problems, such as depression, as well as difficulties with memory and learning. It may also help to protect against arthritis. Vitamin B1 is needed for normal growth in childhood, and for fertility in adult life. In older people it is thought to protect against the development of cataracts.

WHAT IF YOUR INTAKE IS TOO LOW?

Symptoms of vitamin B1 deficiency include fatigue, irritability, mental confusion, forgetfulness and depression. Physically, the nervous system can be damaged and this can cause tingling and numbness in the limbs, as well as weakness and paralysis.

Serious deficiency is unlikely in people who live in developed countries, but it can result in the potentially fatal disease beri-beri, the principal symptoms of which are neuritis and heart failure. Little vitamin B1 is stored in the body so foods that contain it should be eaten every day.

WATER-SOLUBLE VITAMINS

AVAILABILITY IN FOOD

Vitamin B1 is present in many foods, including whole grains and whole-grain products, sunflower seeds, pork, seafood and beans (see also p26). However, it can be lost in cooking, especially when food is boiled or steamed. Intake can be undesirably low if the diet contains too much refined food, such as white flour, rice and sugar.

RIGHT *Try not to overcook sea food to minimize the loss of vitamin B1.*

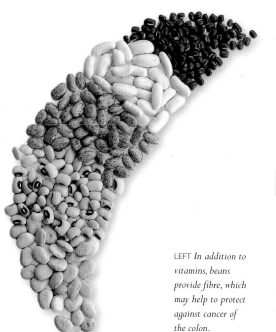

LEFT *In addition to vitamins, beans provide fibre, which may help to protect against cancer of the colon.*

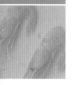

WATER-
SOLUBLE
VITAMINS

CAN TOO MUCH BE TOXIC?

Vitamin B1 is relatively non-toxic and any excess is normally excreted through the kidneys and skin. However, taking large supplements long term (more than 3g a day in an adult) can cause toxicity in the long term.

A GOOD COMBINATION

The absorption of vitamin B1 from the intestine is improved when foods rich in folic acid are eaten at the same time. In the body, it is most effective when the vitamins C and E, and the minerals, manganese and sulphur, are also present.

USING A SUPPLEMENT

If you wish to take a supplement, Vitamin B1 is best taken as part of a balanced B-vitamin tablet or capsule, unless your doctor or nutritional health practitioner advises otherwise.

WHEN EXTRA MAY BE NEEDED

• If you are taking the birth-control pill, diuretics (water pills), digoxin (for heart failure), antacids (for indigestion), or receiving hormone replacement therapy

• If you are on a calorie-restricted diet for any reason. This includes slimmers and older people with small appetites

• If you regularly consume moderate or large amounts of alcohol

• If you suffer from depression or anxiety

• If you pass large volumes of urine

• After surgery or an injury

• During and after an infection

• To prevent air or sea sickness

(Pregnant and breast-feeding women should consult a doctor, midwife, or qualified nutritional therapist before taking any vitamin or mineral supplements.

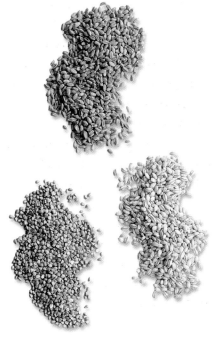

LEFT *Whole cereal grains are nutritious since they are rich in vitamins and minerals, but low in fat.*

VITAMIN B1 AND ALCOHOL

Moderate and heavy drinkers often eat poor diets either because they obtain most of their calories from alcohol or because too much of their money is spent on alcohol.

They are particularly likely to suffer from vitamin B1 deficiency, even if they also eat a good, balanced diet, because the vitamin B1 they consume is of limited use, as alcohol interferes with the way that the vitamin is absorbed into the body from the intestine.

Insufficient vitamin B1 is then available for one of its most important protective roles, which is to break down alcohol into its safe components of carbon dioxide and water, so that it can easily be discharged from the body.

If alcohol cannot be broken down, the body may not be able to withstand its toxic effects and alcohol poisoning can result.

The symptoms of vitamin B1 deficiency may also contribute to the anxiety and confusion often experienced by those who regularly drink too much alcohol.

AVOIDING INSECT BITES

Vitamin B1 is beneficial in many ways, but has an added bonus: it is excreted through the skin and its smell is thought to repel certain biting insects, including mosquitoes and fleas.

RIGHT *Sunflower seeds make an instant snack full of vitamin B1.*

THE B-VITAMINS AND LETHARGY
CARL ROSS

Twenty-one year old Carl had been working in a bar for six months and his regular (though not excessive) alcoholic drinks were beginning to show around his waistline. He began to skip breakfast, but as the weight dropped off he started to feel lethargic and depressed. He was making simple mistakes at work and his boss threatened to sack him.

His mother thought he needed a 'tonic' and gave him a bottle of brewer's yeast tablets. After taking them for a few weeks he began to feel better. At about the same time, he moved in with his girlfriend, who encouraged him to eat breakfast. He improved his diet with a low-sugar breakfast cereal,

choosing one of the brands that are enriched with B-vitamins, and buying nutritious whole-meal bread, yeast extract, and brown rice and pasta. As he began to feel better, he started to cycle to work two or three times a week. Having started a new regime, Carl found his energy levels and mental alertness both improved.

RIGHT *The B-vitamins work together, and many are found in the whole grains and nuts of muesli.*

Vitamin B2
riboflavin

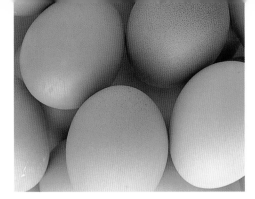

LEFT *Egg dishes provide quick meals that are rich in several B-vitamins.*

Vitamin B2 is the release mechanism that extracts energy from protein, carbohydrate and fat. It helps cells to use oxygen efficiently and is most needed during times of rapid growth, and when protein intake is high. It promotes good vision and healthy hair, skin and nails.

WATER-SOLUBLE VITAMINS

AVAILABILITY IN FOOD

Foods rich in vitamin B2 include liver, cheese, eggs, almonds, and green leafy vegetables (see also p26). Little vitamin B2 is lost from food when it is cooked, but it can be destroyed by light, so foods that contain it should be stored in the dark. In addition, vitamin B2 can be made by bacteria that live in the intestine.

LEFT *Vitamin B2 helps to keep your skin, hair and nails healthy and in good condition.*

WHAT IF YOUR INTAKE IS TOO LOW?

Vitamin B2 is easily absorbed in the small intestine, but only very small quantities are stored in the body, so foods that contain it should be eaten daily. Specific deficiency symptoms include sore, watery eyes that tire easily, burning feet, hair loss, weight loss, and the formation of cataracts. Other symptoms are the same as those of vitamin B6 deficiency, including cracked burning lips, soreness of the tongue, and greasy scaling skin on the face, especially at the sides of the nose.

ABOVE *B-vitamins are added to milk by natural bacteria during the cheese-making process.*

WHEN EXTRA MAY BE NEEDED

• During rapid growth, especially adolescence
• When taking the birth-control pill or receiving hormone replacement therapy
• If you are an older person, especially if you have a small appetite
• If you regularly consume moderate or large amounts of alcohol, or smoke
• During pregnancy and lactation
• While taking antibiotics
• During times of particular stress or excessive activity

LEFT *Store lettuces away from direct light to preserve their vitamin B2 content.*

• When you are on a calorie-restricted diet for any reason (this includes slimmers and older people with small appetites) *(Pregnant and breast-feeding women should consult a doctor, midwife, or qualified nutritional therapist before taking any vitamin or mineral supplements.)*

CAN TOO MUCH BE TOXIC?

There are no known toxic effects of vitamin B2, but excessive supplementation should be avoided as this may cause other B-vitamins to be lost in the urine. Supplements of vitamin B2 can cause yellow discoloration of the urine; this is normal.

A GOOD COMBINATION

Vitamin B2 enhances the activity of vitamin B6 and, if supplements are taken, the dosage of these two vitamins should be about the same. The B-vitamins are more effective when vitamin C is present.

USING A SUPPLEMENT

If you wish to take a supplement, vitamin B2 is best taken as part of a balanced B-vitamin tablet or capsule, unless your doctor or nutritional health practitioner advises otherwise.

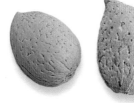

LEFT *Almonds make a tasty snack that is rich in B-vitamins. They also contain less fat than most other nuts.*

SCRAMBLED EGGS, TOAST AND MUSHROOMS

Beat fatigue with food rich in B-vitamins

SERVES **1**

2 eggs, beaten together, seasoned with pepper if desired
1 slice of wholemeal bread
yeast extract
30g (1oz) butter or margarine
60g (2oz) mushrooms, wiped and sliced
freshly chopped parsley

METHOD

Melt half the butter over a low heat and add the mushrooms. Cover and allow them to cook slowly over a low heat. Make the toast and spread with yeast extract. Keep warm.

Melt remaining butter. Do not brown, but when foaming, pour in the eggs and stir briskly to prevent them from sticking to the pan.

Remove eggs from heat when cooked to your taste, and serve on the toast. Garnish with the parsley (contains abundant vitamin C, which enhances the action of the B-vitamins). Serve the mushrooms as a side dish.

WATER-
SOLUBLE
VITAMINS

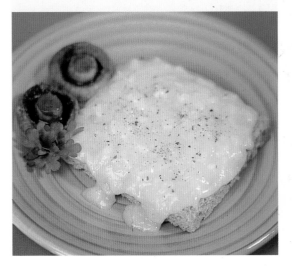

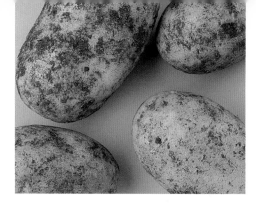

LEFT *Potatoes are filling, fat-free and contain a good supply of B-vitamins and fibre.*

Vitamin B3
niacin

Vitamin B3 helps to break down protein, fat and carbohydrate into the simpler substances needed for the release of energy. It stimulates the circulation, reduces cholesterol levels, and helps in the creation of several hormones, including cortisone and the sex hormones. As well as enhancing normal brain function, vitamin B3 keeps the skin and digestive tract healthy, and is thought to have a role in protecting against cancer.

AVAILABILITY IN FOOD

Vitamin B3 is derived from two compounds: nicotinic acid and niacinamide. Both forms are easily absorbed from the small intestine and have broadly similar actions, although nicotinic acid, in high doses, appears to lower cholesterol.

Vitamin B3 is readily obtainable from nuts, pig's liver, soy flour, wheat, peanut butter and potatoes (see also p26). There is little or no loss in cooking, but up to 90 per cent can be lost from whole grains when they are milled. Food manufacturers often add vitamin B3 to their products to replace this loss.

WHAT IF YOUR INTAKE IS TOO LOW?

Even if the diet contains inadequate vitamin B3, deficiency is unlikely as B3 can be manufactured in the body, provided the diet is otherwise adequate (see Producing your own vitamin B3, p18). If the diet is extremely poor over a long period mental changes, such as irritability, loss of memory and confusion can occur. The skin develops an unpleasant, dry roughness, particularly on the areas exposed to the sun. The tongue becomes painful and cracked, and there are digestive upsets including diarrhoea and loss of appetite. These are the symptoms of pellagra, which can be fatal if left untreated.

WHEN EXTRA MAY BE NEEDED

• If you regularly consume moderate or large amounts of alcohol

• If you do not eat enough protein *(Pregnant and breast-feeding women should consult a doctor, midwife, or qualified nutritional therapist before taking any vitamin or mineral supplements.)*

LEFT *Eat nuts when freshly shelled, as the shells are nature's way of preserving the B-vitamins.*

LEFT *Wholemeal flour is a rich, universally available and economic source of B-vitamins.*

also cause the blood pressure to drop. In younger people, a lower dose (50mg three times a day) to treat or prevent chilblains, can also cause a fall in blood pressure.

To be safe, experts recommend that if you have any medical condition you should consult your doctor before taking vitamin B3 supplements in excess of 50mg per day.

CAN TOO MUCH BE TOXIC?

High doses of nicotinic acid (up to 6g a day) can reduce cholesterol levels and have also been used to clear the body of organic poisons, such as certain pesticides. However, since high doses can also cause liver damage, they should only be taken under medical supervision. Fortunately, the liver heals itself when the high intake of nicotinic acid is reduced.

If taken in excess of about 200mg, nicotinic acid, but not nicotinamide, dilates the blood vessels in the skin and produces flushing. It can

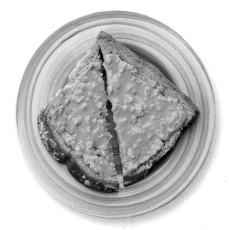

ABOVE *A slice of wholemeal bread with peanut butter gives up to 25 per cent of a 10-year-old's daily needs of vitamin B3.*

WATER-SOLUBLE VITAMINS

VITAMIN B3 AND MENTAL ALERTNESS
JAMIE TAYLOR

After his wife died, his family began to be increasingly worried about Jamie Taylor. He'd always liked a few drinks after work, but he began spending more time in the bar and seemed to be subsisting on a diet of white bread and jam. Although he was still only in his early 70s, he had to be taken home several times when he was found wandering about the village at odd hours, often not properly dressed. When he also began to suffer regular diarrhoea, his daughter discussed his condition with his doctor who diagnosed him as having pellagra and admitted him to hospital.

She was amazed when her father recovered completely after doctors prescribed a course of high doses of B-vitamins administered by injection, followed by oral supplements.

To help him get back on his feet, the dietician suggested he attend cookery classes and soon he was taking great pleasure in cooking meals for his daughter and grandchildren.

A GOOD COMBINATION

Vitamin B3 is most effective when the other B-vitamins and vitamin C are also present.

USING A SUPPLEMENT

If you wish to take a supplement, vitamin B3 is best taken as part of a balanced B-vitamin tablet or capsule, unless your doctor or nutritional health practitioner advises otherwise. If vitamin C is also present it helps to prevent vitamin B3 from being chemically degraded.

BELOW *Milk is a good source of B-vitamins, but adults should drink it skimmed or semi-skimmed to avoid excessive animal fat.*

WATER-
SOLUBLE
VITAMINS

PRODUCING YOUR OWN
VITAMIN B3

Ample vitamin B3 is available for those who eat animal protein as part of a well-balanced diet that contains adequate amounts of vitamin C, iron, and vitamins B1, B2 and B6. These nutrients are the raw materials that can be used by the body to make its own supply of vitamin B3 from an amino acid called tryptophan. This amino acid is abundantly present in both milk and eggs.

Vegans, however, have to take greater care to eat foods that contain sufficient vitamin B3, as plant proteins can be deficient in the amino acid tryptophan as well as being poor sources of vitamin B3. An example is sweetcorn (corn, maize). This grain is deficient in tryptophan and only contains a limited amount of vitamin B3 and that limited amount is in a form that cannot be used by the body without special treatment. Native American Indians knew that pre-treating sweetcorn (corn, maize) by soaking it in ash water prevented the onset of the disease that is now known as pellagra. However, poor white immigrants to the United States in the late nineteenth and early twentieth centuries did not know this and, since their diet consisted largely of untreated cornmeal, the immigrants developed pellagra. In fact, the resulting skin changes of early pellagra are what gave rise to the expression 'rednecks' which became a general term to describe these immigrant field workers.

Vitamin B5
pantothenic acid

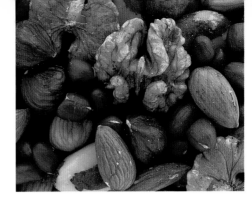

LEFT *Nuts are best eaten raw as some of the B-vitamins are lost during the roasting process.*

Vitamin B5 is an anti-stress vitamin and has a particular role in supporting the adrenal glands as they secrete cortisone and other hormones. These hormones enhance the metabolism generally, aiding the body to overcome allergies and maintain healthy skin, muscles and nerves. Vitamin B5 is thought to reduce skin wrinkles and may delay greying of the hair. Like so many other B-vitamins, it also helps to release energy from food.

AVAILABILITY IN FOOD

Vitamin B5 is widely available in many foods, including pig's liver, fresh nuts, wheat germ, pulses and eggs (see also p26). It can be lost during food preparation, especially in dry heat cooking such as roasting, and during milling when more than 50 per cent of the vitamin B5 naturally occurring in wheat can be lost. It is destroyed when exposed to acids, such as vinegar, or alkalis, such as baking soda. Fortunately, the intestinal bacteria are capable of supplementing the diet with vitamin B5.

WHAT IF YOUR INTAKE IS TOO LOW?

As vitamin B5 is widely available in both plant and animal foods severe, naturally occurring deficiency has not been observed and as yet no recommendation for minimum daily allowances have been made. However, when volunteers were fed a diet low in vitamin B5 they developed many symptoms, including fatigue, headache, dizziness, numbness and tingling, muscle weakness, mood swings, and digestive disturbances.

Mild symptoms of fatigue, digestive problems, frequent infections and worsening of any allergic conditions can develop when intake of vitamin B5 is relatively low, as it can in those who eat a 'fast-food' diet that includes a high proportion of refined sugar and flours.

Teenagers who are growing rapidly as well as eating this type of processed food are more likely to develop symptoms if they are also taking tetracycline antibiotics for acne. Antibiotics can alter the intestinal bacteria and limit their ability to synthesize extra supplies of vitamin B5 within the body.

WATER-SOLUBLE VITAMINS

RIGHT *Eating broccoli, a rich source of B5, is also thought to reduce the risk of cancer.*

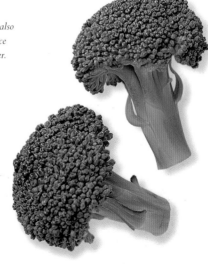

WHEN EXTRA MAY BE NEEDED

- When your lifestyle is very stressful
- If you are prone to allergies
- If your diet consists mostly of processed foods
- If you regularly consume moderate or large amounts of alcohol

(Pregnant and breast-feeding women should consult a doctor, midwife, or qualified nutritional therapist before taking any vitamin or mineral supplements.)

CAN TOO MUCH BE TOXIC?

Vitamin B5 does not appear to be toxic, but digestive disturbances, including diarrhoea, can result from very high doses of around 10g a day. Daily doses of 1,500mg taken over a long period of time can cause excessive sensitivity of the teeth.

A GOOD COMBINATION

Vitamin B5 is most effective when the other B-vitamins, are present together with vitamin C, and the minerals, calcium and sulphur.

USING A SUPPLEMENT

If you wish to take a supplement, vitamin B5 is best taken as part of a balanced B-vitamin tablet or capsule, unless your doctor or nutritional health practitioner advises otherwise.

ABOVE *Lentils are a good source of B-vitamins as well as soluble and insoluble fibre.*

PANCAKE SCONES

Beat fatigue with food rich in B-vitamins

MAKES ABOUT 12 SCONES
170g (8oz) whole-grain flour of your choice (e.g. wheat, rye, oats, millet, barley, buckwheat)
2 level teaspoons of baking powder
1 tablespoon of honey (optional)
1 tablespoon of olive oil
1 egg
125ml (6fl oz) milk, plus extra as needed
30–60g (1–2oz) finely chopped walnuts (optional)

METHOD
Mix all the ingredients, except for the walnuts (if used), together in a food processor or blender. Add more milk to make a consistency similar to thick cream, and then stir in the walnuts.

Heat and lightly grease a frying pan and drop one or more single tablespoons of the mixture onto the hot surface. When bubbles form on the tops of the scones, flip them over and cook the other side. When cooked, either cool the scones on a rack or keep them warm at a very low temperature in the oven while you cook the rest of the mixture, re-greasing the pan between batches.

Serve with butter, peanut butter, yeast extract, honey or jam.

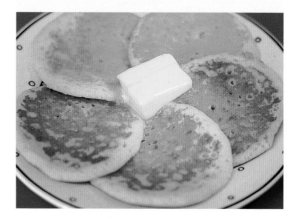

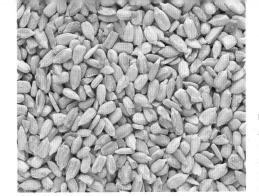

LEFT *Sunflower seeds are packed with nutrition, including the B-vitamins, especially when eaten raw.*

Vitamin B6
pyridoxine

Vitamin B6 is a very hard-working vitamin that is probably best known for its ability to balance hormonal changes in women (see Vitamin B6 and women, p23). In addition, it is probably the most important of the B-vitamins for the immune system, enabling the body to protect itself from infection and, possibly, to inhibit the growth of cancer cells. It aids the production of new cells, including those that make up the immune system and the red blood cells.

Like so many of the B-vitamins, vitamin B6 enables the body to process dietary protein, fat, sugars and starches effectively, and may help in weight control. It helps to control mood and behaviour, and is one of the vitamins that nutritionists recommend for children who are hyperactive or have learning difficulties. Vitamin B6 is also needed to keep skin healthy and it may help to prevent conditions such as dandruff, eczema and psoriasis.

AVAILABILITY IN FOOD

Vitamin B6 is readily absorbed into the body, but vitamin B2 and magnesium are both needed to convert it into its active form. Fortunately, these are both found in many of the same foods that contain vitamin B6, such as liver, kidney, sunflower seeds, wheat germ, walnuts, beans and eggs (see also p26). The production of the active form of vitamin B6 is also aided by exercise.

Although vitamin B6 is present in many foods, it can be destroyed by sunlight, so foods that contain it should be stored in the dark. It is lost during cooking and when foods are processed, for example during milling. The bacteria in the intestine can supplement the diet by manufacturing extra supplies. Vitamin B6 is not stored in the body, and foods containing it should be eaten several times a day as it is rapidly lost in the urine.

WHAT IF YOUR INTAKE IS TOO LOW?

As vitamin B6 has such a wide range of activity, the whole body is involved if deficiency occurs and many of the symptoms are similar to those seen when vitamins B2 and B3 are lacking. Indeed, vitamin B6 is essential for the body to make its own vitamin B3 (see p19).

BELOW *Pork contains both vitamins B2 and B6, which complement each other well.*

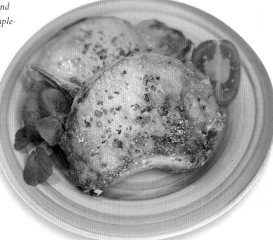

WATER-SOLUBLE VITAMINS

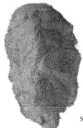

In addition to the symptoms specific to women (see Vitamin B6 and women, p23), vitamin B6 deficiency can cause irritability, nervousness, insomnia, weakness and even convulsions. Skin changes include dermatitis and acne. The nails may be ridged and the tongue inflamed. Asthma and other allergies may develop, as may anaemia. Bone changes include osteoporosis and arthritis, and kidney stones can occur.

WHEN EXTRA MAY BE NEEDED

• When taking the birth-control pill or receiving hormone replacement therapy
• If you suffer from pre-menstrual symptoms
• During pregnancy and when breast feeding
• If you suffer from psychological problems, such as depression or anxiety
• When on a calorie-restricted diet for any reason (this includes slimmers and older people with small appetites)
• If you consume moderate or large amounts of alcohol
• If you eat a high-protein diet, or a diet high in sugar and processed foods
• If you are allergic to monosodium glutamate or tartrazine

(Pregnant and breast-feeding women should consult a doctor, midwife, or qualified nutritional therapist before taking any vitamin or mineral supplements.)

CAN TOO MUCH BE TOXIC?

Supplements should not exceed 50mg per day unless prescribed by a doctor. You may have vivid dreams if you take supplements in the late evening.

Extreme supplementation (over 2,000mg a day) could cause neurological damage. If you are taking levo-dopa, which is prescribed for Parkinson's disease, you should not take vitamin B6 supplements as they can inactivate it. (This does not occur with 'Sinemet'.)

A GOOD COMBINATION

Vitamin B6 should always be taken with other B-vitamins, and at broadly the same dose as vitamin B2, needed by the body to convert vitamin B6 into its active form. Because vitamin B6 has such as wide range of action, a number of other nutrients are needed to enable the body to make the best use of it, including vitamin C, the minerals magnesium, sodium, potassium and zinc, and the fatty acid, linoleic acid (see vitamin F).

USING A SUPPLEMENT

If you wish to take a supplement, vitamin B6 is best taken as part of a balanced B-vitamin tablet or capsule, unless your doctor or nutritional health practitioner advises otherwise. Ideally, vitamin B6 supplements should be divided into more than one dose because any excess is rapidly lost in the urine.

LEFT *Boost your B-vitamin intake with a tablespoon of brewer's yeast dissolved in a glass of tomato juice.*

WATER-SOLUBLE VITAMINS

LEFT *Vitamin B6 can reduce the symptoms caused by the monthly changes in women's hormone levels.*

RIGHT *An egg at breakfast time will get your B-vitamin intake for the day off to a good start.*

VITAMIN B6 AND WOMEN

Vitamin B6 has a particular importance for women, as it seems able to reduce the symptoms that are caused when hormone levels change. Unfortunately, many women do not eat enough foods that are rich in vitamin B6, and are prone to a variety of symptoms at different stages of life, such as:

• Pre-menstrual fluid retention causing breast tenderness and emotional symptoms

• Pre-menstrual acne

• Period pains

• Nausea and sickness in early pregnancy

(*Note: although many women do take moderate doses of vitamin B6 supplements during the first three months of pregnancy, its absolute safety has not been established, and individual advice should be sought.*)

• High blood pressure, fluid retention and poor control of blood sugar in later pregnancy

• Emotional symptoms (mood swings, depression and loss of sex drive) when taking the birth-control pill or hormone replacement therapy.

In the short term, taking vitamin B6 supplements will often help to alleviate these symptoms. However, it is also important to improve your diet because the B-vitamins occur in the same foods, and deficiency in one of the B-vitamins often means that others will be in short supply as well.

WATER-SOLUBLE VITAMINS

KEEP YOUR HEART HEALTHY

There is growing evidence that vitamin B6 and folic acid can work together to reduce the risk of heart attacks. They enable the body to break down excessive levels of homocysteine, a substance that is known to predispose to heart attacks. Good sources of both vitamins are brewer's yeast, green leafy vegetables and foods made from whole wheat or oats. In addition, a number of breakfast cereals are now fortified with these vitamins.

VITAMIN B6 AND PRE-MENSTRUAL SYMPTOMS
TRISHA CONNOR

Trisha Connor, a 31-year-old working mother of three, consulted her doctor for a repeat prescription of the birth-control pill. She mentioned that, before her periods, her breasts were very painful and that she would often cry at-work without any particular reason. Her doctor agreed that she should consult a nutritional therapist who gave her dietary advice and suggested some vitamin supplements that included vitamin B6.

After a few months, Trisha's symptoms had improved and she felt much better. She had also noticed that, since she had changed the diet for the whole family by including more whole grains, fruit and vegetables, her husband seemed to have more energy and her children had been less quarrelsome.

Folic acid

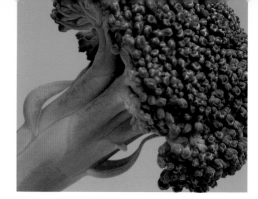

LEFT *Eat green vegetables, such as broccoli, every day to ensure that your body has an ample supply of folic acid.*

WATER-
SOLUBLE
VITAMINS

Folic acid, which is sometimes known as folacin or folate, works with vitamin B12 to protect the nervous system, especially the developing nervous system of the foetus, and to manufacture red blood cells. Folic acid stimulates appetite and aids digestion, as well as improving mental and emotional health by its effect on the nervous system. It is needed for healthy skin and hair.

AVAILABILITY IN FOOD

The best sources of folic acid are fresh green leafy vegetables such as spinach and broccoli. However, it is also found in fruits, starchy vegetables, whole grains and liver (see also p26). Folic acid is commonly deficient in the modern Western diet, as light, heat, and storage at room temperature can easily destroy it. Fortunately, the intestinal bacteria can manufacture folic acid, and stores in the liver can last for up to six months.

WHAT IF YOUR INTAKE IS TOO LOW?

Early symptoms are fatigue, apathy or irritability, loss of appetite, acne, a sore tongue, and cracking of the corners of the mouth (this also results from deficiencies of iron, or vitamins B2 or B6). Anaemia develops somewhat later, and in the longer term there are increased risks of osteoporosis (see p61), heart attacks if vitamin B6 is also low (see p23), and certain cancers, especially of the bowel and cervix.

WHEN EXTRA MAY BE NEEDED

• During pregnancy and lactation
• If the diet contains insufficient fresh food
• While taking the birth-control pill, long-term antibiotics, or hormone replacement therapy
• By children if they drink goats' milk instead of cows' milk
• During stress or illness
• If you have a moderate to high alcohol consumption
• If you have psoriasis
(Pregnant and breast-feeding women should consult a doctor, midwife, or qualified nutritional therapist before taking any vitamin or mineral supplements.)

LEFT *Wholemeal bread, especially if spread with yeast extract, provides a quick snack rich in B-vitamins.*

CAN TOO MUCH BE TOXIC?

More than 15mg of folic acid taken regularly can cause digestive upset, insomnia and loss of energy. You should consult your doctor before taking folic acid supplements if you take medication for epilepsy, as it alters the way these drugs work, or if you are at risk of pernicious anaemia (see p27–28). This condition tends to occur within families and in older people, and folic acid supplementation should be avoided as it can cause permanent damage to the nerves.

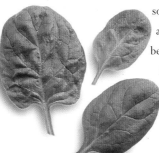

ABOVE *Folic acid, which was first discovered in spinach, is needed to make red blood cells.*

A GOOD COMBINATION

Folic acid is most effective when the other B-vitamins, especially B12 and B6, and vitamin C are present.

USING A SUPPLEMENT

If you wish to take a supplement, folic acid is best taken as part of a balanced B-vitamin tablet or capsule, unless your doctor or nutritional health practitioner advises otherwise.

FOLIC ACID AND PREGNANCY

All women are advised to take a small supplement of folic acid during pregnancy to reduce the risk of the baby being born with spina bifida or other serious congenital defects of the nervous system.

During their childbearing years, women should eat a diet rich in folic acid at all times, and ask their doctors about a supplement before they are planning to get pregnant, or as soon as possible if they are already pregnant. A baby will benefit from a good supply of folic acid, particularly early on in the pregnancy

Adequate folic acid intake is also thought to reduce the likelihood of toxaemia of pregnancy, of haemorrhage and of premature labour.

In addition, it appears to reduce the incidence of 'restless leg syndrome' in late pregnancy, and to enhance the production of breast milk after delivery.

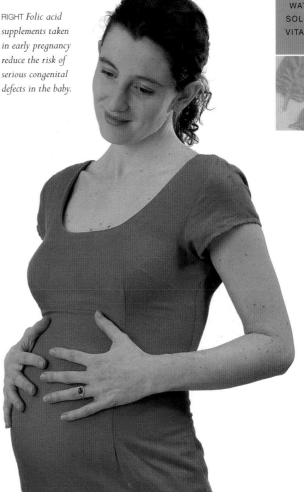

RIGHT *Folic acid supplements taken in early pregnancy reduce the risk of serious congenital defects in the baby.*

WATER-SOLUBLE VITAMINS

Vitamin B-rich foods

FOODS RICH IN VITAMINS B1, B2, B3, B5 AND FOLIC ACID.

These B vitamins work together, and are often found in the same foods and natural supplements, some of which are listed here.

	B1 Thiamine	B2 Riboflavine	B3 Niacin	B5 Pantothenic acid	B6 Pyridoxine	Folic acid
	mg per 100g (3½ oz)	mg per 100g (3½ oz)	mg per 100g (3½ oz)	mg per 100g (3½ oz)	mg per 100g (3½ oz)	mcg per 100gm (3½ oz)
Brewer's yeast [1]	15.6	4.3	38	4.2	9.5	240
Yeast extract [2]	5.8	7	160	1.2	0.1	2,500
Blackstrap molasses [3]	0.1	0.2	2	0.5	0.27	10
DAIRY						
Cheddar cheese	0.04	0.5	6.22	0.3	0.08	20
Egg (raw)	0.09	0.47	3.68	1.8	0.11	25
Milk	0.04	0.19	0.86	0.35	0.04	5
MEAT						
Pork	0.6	0.2	10	1	0.3	5
Lamb	0.1	0.2	10	0.5	0.18	3
Liver	0.27	2.5	17	6.7	0.6	300
Kidney	0.35	2.1	13	3.8	0.27	60
GRAINS, PULSES & NUTS						
Brown rice	0.34	0.04	4.5	1	0.5	16
White rice	0.08	0.03	3	0.6	0.3	29
Rye flour	0.4	0.22	2.6	1	0.35	78
Wholemeal flour	0.46	0.08	8.1	0.8	0.5	57
Wheat germ	1.45	0.61	11.1	1.7	0.95	330
Soya flour (full fat)	0.75	0.31	10.6	1.8	0.57	400
Lentils (cooked)	0.11	0.03	1.6	0.31	0.11	5
Hazel nuts	0.4	0	3.1	1.15	0.55	72
Peanuts fresh	0.9	0.1	21.3	2.7	0.5	110
roasted and salted	0.23	0.1	21.3	2.1	0.4	0
Walnuts	0.3	0.13	3	0.9	0.73	66
VEGETABLES & FRUIT						
Avocado	0.1	0.1	1.8	1.07	0.42	66
Broccoli raw	0.1	0.3	1.6	1	0.21	130
boiled	0.06	0.2	1.2	0.7	0.13	120
French beans	0.04	0.07	0.5	0.07	0.06	28
Raw Savoy cabbage	0.06	0.05	0.8	0.21	0.16	90
Raw white cabbage	0.06	0.05	0.6	0.21	0.16	26
Honeydew melon	0.05	0.03	0.5	0.23	0.07	30
Raw mushrooms	0.1	0.4	4.6	2	0.1	23
Potatoes (baked with skin)	0.08	0.03	1.5	0.16	0.14	8
Plums (raw)	0.05	0.03	0.6	0.15	0.05	3
Spinach	0.07	0.15	1.8	0.21	0.18	140

[1] **Brewer's yeast** Although brewer's yeast was originally a by-product of the brewing industry, it is now specifically produced as a food supplement, which can be bought at health food shops. It is astonishingly rich in nutrients, being a source of good quality-protein, many minerals, including iron, copper, chromium and selenium, and excellent concentrations of B-vitamins. It also contains glucose tolerance factor (GTF), which helps to normalize blood sugar levels in diabetes and hypoglycaemia (low blood sugar), and may help to moderate the pre-menstrual craving for starchy and sweet foods that many women experience. If you wish to take brewer's yeast as a food supplement, start with a low dose and gradually increase as the body adapts to it. It is available in tablet, flake or powder form. If you are intolerant of yeast or prone to recurrent infections with candida (thrush), avoid supplements.

[2] **Yeast extract** Various yeast extracts are available as proprietary spreads, and can be bought at supermarkets and health-food shops. They are a rich source of the B-vitamins, but avoid them if you are intolerant of yeast or prone to candida (thrush) infections.

[3] **Blackstrap molasses** Blackstrap molasses is the concentrated syrup that is left after refined sugar has been removed from sugar cane. It can be bought at health-food shops and is a rich source of B-vitamins and minerals, including copper, magnesium, phosphorus, iron, calcium, potassium, magnesium, chromium, manganese, molybdenum and zinc. One tablespoon of molasses contains over 100mg of calcium (as much as a glass of milk) and 3mg of iron (as much as 60g (2oz) of liver).

When taken as a supplement, up to about one tablespoonful is adequate for adults (half of this for children). It can be eaten instead of jam or jelly, used in cakes, such as gingerbread, or even in savoury dishes such as Boston baked beans. If taken regularly, it is reported to be beneficial for eczema, arthritis, anaemia, fatigue, stomach ulcers and constipation. Although most of the sugar has been removed, molasses can still cause tooth decay and teeth should be cleaned after eating it.

Vitamin B12
cobolamin

LEFT *Vitamin B12 occurs in food from animals, including egg yolks.*

Vitamin B12 has been termed the 'energy' vitamin and the scientific support for this definition is gradually growing. Its major well-established functions, however, are in the manufacture of red blood cells and the maintenance of healthy nerves.

In childhood, vitamin B12 is needed to stimulate appetite, promote growth, especially of the nervous system, and to release energy from food. It has a reputation for rejuvenating old people physically by providing energy, and mentally by preventing mental deterioration and speeding up thought processes. Throughout life it appears to help to overcome infection and provide protection against allergies and cancer.

AVAILABILITY IN FOOD

Significant amounts of vitamin B12 are found only in foods from animal sources, especially liver, oily fish and egg yolk. Bacteria in the intestine can manufacture it, but it is not known to what extent vitamin B12 produced in this way can be absorbed and used. Although there have been claims that vegetarian products, such as tempeh, miso, some seed sprouts and spirulina contain good supplies of vitamin B12, this has not been confirmed by independent analysis. Some vitamin B12 is present in sea vegetables (see Sea weed as food, p83), but its chemical make-up is slightly different from animal B12, and it is not certain how active it is. Various studies have shown that vitamin B12 can be seriously deficient in children who are given a strict vegan or macrobiotic diet.

WHAT IF YOUR INTAKE IS TOO LOW?

Vitamin B12 is only needed in very small amounts, perhaps less than 1mcg a day, and the liver can store several years' supply. As a result, the most common reason for vitamin B12 deficiency is failure of the body to absorb it because of changes in digestion, rather than from any dietary insufficiency. Vitamin B12 deficiency

WATER-SOLUBLE VITAMINS

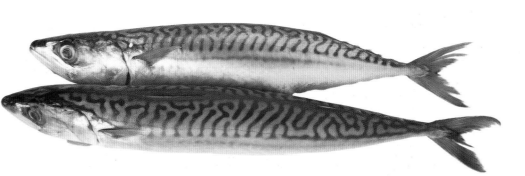

RIGHT *Oily fish, such as mackerel, should be eaten at least once or twice each week.*

causes an extremely serious condition called pernicious anaemia, when there are too few red blood cells and the spinal cord and other nerve cells can become permanently damaged. Symptoms include pallor, shortness of breath, weakness, fatigue, mental slowness, numbness, tingling and shooting pains in the limbs, clumsiness and difficulty in walking. Untreated, it can be fatal.

LEFT *Chicken is a source of vitamin B12 that is also low in fat.*

WHEN EXTRA MAY BE NEEDED

• If you eat a strict vegan diet

• If you are an elderly person

• During pregnancy and when breast feeding

• If you regularly consume moderate or large amounts of alcohol

• If you regularly take laxatives or antacid preparations

(Pregnant and breast-feeding women should consult a doctor, midwife, or qualified nutritional therapist before taking any vitamin or mineral supplements.)

CAN TOO MUCH BE TOXIC?

There is no evidence that vitamin B12 is toxic when taken by mouth as the body does not absorb enough. If administered by injection, too much vitamin B12 can cause skin problems, but these will quickly go away once the injections have been discontinued.

A GOOD COMBINATION

Vitamin B12 is more effective in the presence of the other B-vitamins, vitamin C, iron, calcium, sodium and potassium.

USING A SUPPLEMENT

If you wish to take a supplement, vitamin B12 is best taken as part of a balanced B-vitamin tablet or capsule, unless your doctor or nutritional health practitioner advises otherwise.

Supplements prescribed by doctors for the treatment of pernicious anaemia are usually administered by injection.

GOOD FOOD SOURCES OF VITAMIN B12

mcg per 100g (3½oz)	
Pig's liver	25
Fatty fish	5
White fish	2
Beef	2
Eggs	2
Cheese	1
Chicken	0.5
Milk	0.3

Biotin

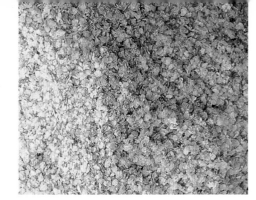

Biotin (occasionally known as vitamin H) helps the body to make best use of fats and proteins, and to maintain a steady level of sugar in the blood. It keeps the skin and hair healthy, and may enhance the performance of athletes.

RIGHT *Milk promotes healthy hair and skin.*

AVAILABILITY IN FOODS

Small amounts of biotin are found in brewer's yeast, meat, nuts and dairy products, and bacteria in the intestine make up any dietary shortfall. Biotin is not lost in cooking.

WHAT IF YOUR INTAKE IS TOO LOW?

Provided the calorie intake is adequate, biotin deficiency is uncommon. However, raw egg white contains a substance that can bind with biotin in the stomach and prevent its absorption into the body. People who eat large amounts of raw eggs develop nausea, fatigue, dermatitis and depression.

WHEN EXTRA MAY BE NEEDED

• During pregnancy and lactation

• If you take long-term antibiotics

• If you are on a restricted and very low-calorie diet

(Pregnant and breast-feeding women should consult a doctor, midwife, or qualified nutritional therapist before taking any vitamin or mineral supplements.)

CAN TOO MUCH BE TOXIC?

There are no known toxic symptoms, probably because excess is easily lost in the urine and faeces.

A GOOD COMBINATION

Biotin should always be taken as part of a general B-vitamin supplement. It is most effective when vitamin C and sulphur are present.

USING A SUPPLEMENT

Biotin is best taken as part of a balanced B-vitamin tablet or capsule, unless your doctor or nutritional health practitioner advises otherwise.

WATER-SOLUBLE VITAMINS

GOOD FOOD SOURCES OF BIOTIN	
mcg per 100g (3½oz)	
Dried brewer's yeast	80
Pig's kidney	32
Yeast extract	27
Eggs	25
Wheat germ	12
Wholemeal bread	6
Fatty fish	5
Milk, cheese and yoghurt	2

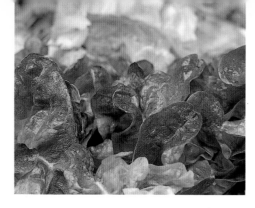

LEFT *Many vitamins, including choline, are lost from green vegetables that are stored for too long.*

Choline

Choline helps to control weight and cholesterol levels, to prevent gallstones and to keep cell membranes healthy. It is essential for the nervous system, aids memory and learning, and may help to fight viral infections, including the hepatitis viruses and AIDS.

WATER-
SOLUBLE
VITAMINS

AVAILABILITY IN FOOD

Choline is widely available in foods, including soy products and leafy vegetables. It can be lost in cooking, long-term storage and food processing.

WHAT IF YOUR INTAKE IS TOO LOW?

Dietary insufficiency is very rare, but it can cause diseases of the liver and kidney, raised cholesterol and high blood pressure.

WHEN EXTRA MAY BE NEEDED

- If you regularly consume moderate or high amounts of alcohol
- If you eat large amounts of refined sugar
- If you are taking large amounts of nicotinic acid to control cholesterol levels (see p17)

    (Pregnant and breast-feeding women should consult a doctor, midwife, or qualified nutritional therapist before taking any vitamin or mineral supplements.)

CAN TOO MUCH BE TOXIC?

Excessive supplements may cause nausea, depression and aggravate pre-existing epilepsy. Too much choline can lead to the body exuding a fishy odour, when supplementation should be stopped.

A GOOD COMBINATION

Choline should always be taken with the other B-vitamins and in about the same dose as inosital as these vitamins work together to maintain cell membranes. It is most effective when vitamin A and linoleic acid (see vitamin F, p51) are present.

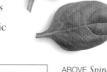

USING A SUPPLEMENT

If you wish to take a supplement, choline is best taken as part of a balanced B-vitamin tablet or capsule, unless your doctor or nutritional health practitioner advises otherwise.

ABOVE *Spinach should be eaten when it is young, and either raw or lightly cooked.*

GOOD FOOD SOURCES OF CHOLINE

mg per 100gm (3½oz)	
Beef heart	1,720
Egg yolk	1,700
Beef steak	600
Wheat germ	500
Oatflakes	240
Nuts	220

Inosital

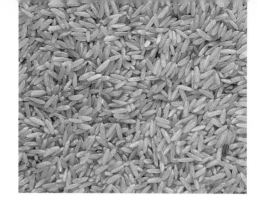

LEFT *The inosital and the fibre in brown rice act together to keep the bowel regular.*

Inosital has a particular role in the maintenance of cell membranes, especially those of the brain, bone marrow, eye and intestines. Cell membranes control the contents of the cells, enabling them to function effectively. Inosital promotes healthy skin and hair growth. It helps to control oestrogen levels and may help to prevent breast lumps.

AVAILABILITY IN FOOD

Inosital is widely available in animal food and plants including fresh fruit, cereals and pulses. In plants it occurs as phytic acid which can prevent the absorption of minerals by binding with them. To prevent this, cereals and pulses should be cooked or sprouted. The intestinal bacteria can also manufacture inosital and as the body normally contains stores, daily intake is not essential.

WHAT IF YOUR INTAKE IS TOO LOW?

Eczema, hair loss, constipation, and raised cholesterol may occur, but deficiency of inosital is rare.

WHEN EXTRA BE NEEDED

• If you regularly drink more than two cups of coffee a day
• If you are taking long-term antibiotics

(Pregnant and breast-feeding women should consult a doctor, midwife, or qualified nutritional therapist before taking any vitamin or mineral supplements.)

CAN TOO MUCH BE TOXIC?

There is no known toxicity.

A GOOD COMBINATION

Inosital should be taken in combination with the other B-vitamins, and in much the same dose as choline. Vitamins C and E and linoleic acid (see vitamin F, p51) may enhance its function if they are taken at the same time.

USING A SUPPLEMENT

If you wish to take a supplement, inosital is best taken as part of a balanced B-vitamin tablet or capsule, unless your doctor or nutritional health practitioner advises otherwise.

WATER-SOLUBLE VITAMINS

GOOD FOOD SOURCES OF INOSITAL	
mg per 100gm (3½oz)	
Beef heart	1,600
Wheat germ	690
Liver	340
Brown rice	330
Oatflakes	320
Nuts	180
Bananas	120

Para-aminobenzoic acid (PABA)

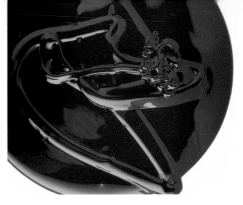

LEFT *Molasses is the vitamin-rich syrup that is left behind after refined sugar has been extracted from sugar cane.*

WATER-
SOLUBLE
VITAMINS

PABA is related to folic acid and acts to improve the way that protein is used in the body. It assists in the formation of red blood cells and enhances the formation of folic acid in the intestine.

PABA's most frequent use is in sunscreen preparations, as it has the ability to protect the skin against excessive ultra-violet light exposure. However, when used above factor 8 it can reduce the ability of the skin to produce vitamin D (see p45). It is said to stimulate hair growth and reverse greying of the hair, but when used to treat grey hair the results have been poor.

AVAILABILITY IN FOODS

PABA is found in molasses, brewer's yeast, liver, whole grains and eggs. In addition, it can be made by the intestinal bacteria. Any excess is stored in the body.

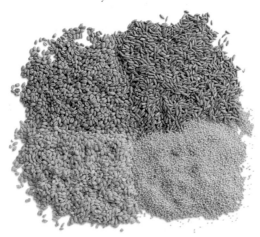

WHAT IF YOUR INTAKE IS TOO LOW?

Deficiency is uncommon, but may result in general fatigue, depression and irritability, and constipation may occur.

WHEN EXTRA MAY BE NEEDED

• If you are taking long-term antibiotics (but PABA reduces the effectiveness of the sulphono-mide antibiotics)

(Pregnant and breast-feeding women should consult a doctor, midwife, or qualified nutritional therapist before taking any vitamin or mineral supplements.)

CAN TOO MUCH BE TOXIC?

PABA can cause nausea, vomiting and skin rashes. It is stored in the body and excessive levels may cause may cause liver damage.

A GOOD COMBINATION

PABA should be taken with other B-vitamins rather than on its own, and it works best in the presence of vitamin C.

USING A SUPPLEMENT

Few nutritional practitioners advise taking a supplement of PABA on its own. It is best taken as part of a balanced B-vitamin tablet or capsule, unless your doctor or nutritional health practitioner advises otherwise.

LEFT *PABA is one of the many B-vitamins that are plentiful in whole grains, but can be lost during milling.*

Vitamin B13
orotic acid

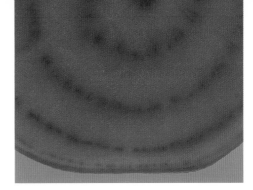

LEFT *Beetroot is a great winter standby that can be eaten either raw or cooked.*

Despite being known as vitamin B13, orotic acid is not really recognized as a vitamin. It helps in the production of genetic material in the cells, and may help after a heart attack.

AVAILABILITY IN FOOD

Orotic acid is found in liquid whey and root vegetables, such as carrots and beets. It is stable to heat.

WHAT IF YOUR INTAKE IS TOO LOW?

Orotic acid is manufactured in the intestine by bacteria in adequate quantities.

WHEN EXTRA MAY BE NEEDED

At present it is not thought to be essential.

CAN TOO MUCH BE TOXIC?

Toxicity has not been reported

USING A SUPPLEMENT

Supplements are not recommended for healthy adults, although doctors may prescribe orotic acid for conditions such as multiple sclerosis and chronic hepatitis.

RIGHT
Even children who hate vegetables may enjoy eating raw carrots.

RIGHT *Add a few seeds to salad for extra food value.*

VALUE-ADDED SALADS

Edible seeds may be small but they are packed with nutritional value, including essential fats (see p51–53). Sprinkle a few over your salads. If you like them crunchy, soak them in water, preferably spring water, for an hour or so beforehand.

• Sunflower seeds contain several B-vitamins, vitamins A, E and D as well as calcium, magnesium, phosphorus, iron, zinc, potassium and iodine.

• Pumpkin seeds contain a mix of B-vitamins and vitamin E as well as zinc, iron, calcium, phosphorus, magnesium and copper.

• Sesame seeds (see also p40 and p53) contain good quality protein and unsaturated fatty acids. They are also a rich source of calcium, magnesium, vitamins A, E and B3.

• Grape seeds contain powerful anti-oxidant substances that are much more effective than vitamin C. If you do not fancy chewing grape seeds, their oil is available for use in salad dressing, or you can obtain the anti-oxidants from a glass of wine. Grape seed extract is also available in capsules as a food supplement, usually marketed as OPCs (oligomeric proanthocyanidins).

WATER-
SOLUBLE
VITAMINS

Vitamin B15
pangamic acid

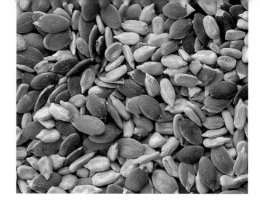

LEFT *Seeds from sunflowers and pumpkins are little power houses, packed with nutritional goodness.*

WATER-
SOLUBLE
VITAMINS

To qualify as a vitamin, a substance must be essential in the diet and, even though pangamic acid is often known as vitamin B15, we do not yet know that it is essential. Much of the research into this substance was conducted in Russia and has not been substantiated in the West.

AVAILABILITY IN FOOD

Pangamic acid occurs naturally in brown rice, brewer's yeast, whole grains, pumpkin seeds and sunflower seeds.

WHAT IF YOUR INTAKE IS TOO LOW?

At present it is not thought to be essential.

WHEN EXTRA MAY BE NEEDED

At present it is not thought to be essential.

CAN TOO MUCH BE TOXIC?

At present there is no evidence of toxicity when pangamic acid is taken in food. However, a substance called dimethylglycine (DMG) is thought to be the active ingredient of pangamic acid, and there is some concern that it might have the ability to cause cancer. Until there has been further research, it would be wise to avoid any product that is labelled pangamic acid, calcium pangamate, DMG or B15.

FAR LEFT *Brewer's yeast should be avoided if you are allergic or sensitive to yeast.*

BELOW *Brown rice is, nutritionally, much superior to white rice.*

BELOW *The pangamic acid in whole grains may help to slow the ageing process.*

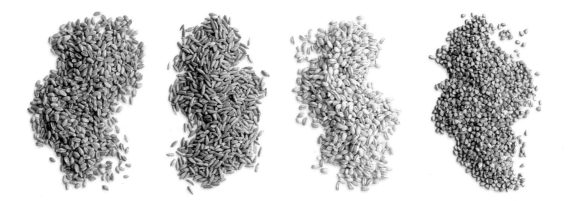

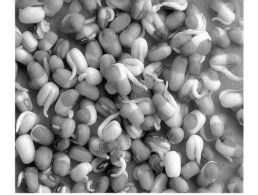

LEFT *Sprouted mung beans do not cause toxicity when eaten in average-sized portions.*

Vitamin B17
laetrile or amygdalin

It is questionable whether vitamin B17 is truly a vitamin. It is said to prevent the growth and spread of cancers but without scientific basis and this use has been outlawed in some countries. Laetrile may help to reduce blood pressure and the pain of arthritis.

AVAILABILITY IN FOOD

Laetrile is present in the kernels of apricots; it is also present to a lesser extent in the kernels of other stone fruit, such as plums, peaches and cherries, and in the pips of apples and nectarines. Laetrile can also be found in sprouting seeds, especially those of mung beans, pictured above right.

WHAT IF YOUR INTAKE IS TOO LOW?

At present it is not thought to be essential

WHEN EXTRA MAY BE NEEDED

At present it is not thought to be essential.

CAN TOO MUCH BE TOXIC?

Vitamin B17 contains cyanide, which is thought to be the cause of toxic symptoms. These include cold sweats, headaches, nausea, blue lips and low blood pressure.

USING A SUPPLEMENT

This is not recommended. The vitamin B17 in sprouted seeds is safe in average-sized portions.

WATER-SOLUBLE VITAMINS

SUPER SPROUTS

Young shoots from recently germinated seeds have been part of the Chinese diet for thousands of years, and with good reason. They are rich in vitamins A, C, D, E, K and the B-vitamins, as well as minerals, such as calcium, phosphorus, potassium, magnesium and iron. They stimulate the appetite and help the body to rid itself of waste products and water. They are said to relieve arthritis, and stomach and duodenal ulcers.

Sprouts from a variety of seeds are now available in supermarkets and health-food stores and can enrich the food value of salads, sandwiches and stir-fries. Try sprouting your own: choose from dried peas, whole lentils, mung beans, chickpeas, radish or other brassica seeds. Soak the seeds in spring water overnight (or up to 24 hours for very large seeds) and drain them. If you do not have a sprouter, place the seeds in a glass jar and tie a piece of muslin over the top. Keep the seeds in a warm, dark place and rinse them in fresh water three times a day, draining well each time. After three to five days they will be ready to use.

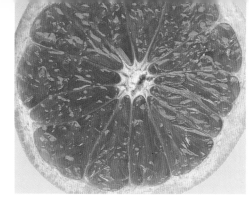

Vitamin C
ascorbic acid

LEFT *Eat plenty of citrus fruit when you have a cold or infection as the vitamins C and P they contain will boost your immune system and help the healing process.*

Vitamin C is essential for the production of collagen, which is a structural protein that holds the body together and is essential for the healing of wounds. Vitamin C is vital for a healthy skin and helps to delay the onset of wrinkles, as well as other age-related disorders such as arthritis. It boosts the immune system, alleviates allergic conditions and enhances the production of several hormones. It is probably the vitamin that is most frequently taken as a supplement.

GOOD FOOD SOURCES OF VITAMIN C

	mg per 100g (3½oz)
Raw red peppers	280
Brussels sprouts	200
Parsley	150
Green peppers (raw)	100
Tomato puree	100
Kiwi fruit (raw)	98
Strawberries (raw)	60
Mange tout peas (stir fried)	52
Raw cabbage	49
Orange juice	33
French fries	11

AVAILABILITY IN FOOD

Vitamin C is found mainly in fresh fruit and vegetables, including citrus fruits, tomatoes, melons, green leafy vegetables and papayas. Very little vitamin C is stored in the body and, as it cannot be manufactured in humans, foods containing it should be eaten every day, preferably at every meal. It is easily lost from food in cooking (see Cooking Tips, p38).

WHAT IF YOUR INTAKE IS TOO LOW?

A wide range of medical problems has been associated with insufficient vitamin C, including increased susceptibility to infections of all types, poor wound-healing and easy bruising, anaemia, asthma, heart disease and psychological problems such as anxiety and depression. Severe deficiency causes the bleeding gums, painful joints, muscle fatigue and dry scaly skin of scurvy, which is fortunately rare nowadays. However, some of these symptoms may occur if you suddenly stop taking high doses of vitamin C supplements: they should be reduced gradually to give the body time to adjust.

WHEN EXTRA MAY BE NEEDED

• During times of stress, or when you are exposed to heavy pollution

BELOW *To benefit from the high quantities of vitamin C in young mange tout peas, eat them raw in a salad or cook them by steaming very briefly.*

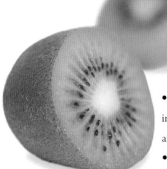

LEFT *Cut the top off a kiwi fruit and eat it like a boiled egg for a vitamin C feast.*

• When you have an infection, especially if you are on antibiotics

• After surgery, or if you have a wound that is slow to heal, such as a leg ulcer

• If you smoke or regularly consume moderate or large amounts of alcohol

• When taking the birth-control pill, anti-histamine medication for allergies, steroids, or receiving hormone replacement therapy

(Pregnant and breast-feeding women should consult a doctor, midwife or qualified nutritional therapist before taking any vitamin or mineral supplement.)

CAN TOO MUCH BE TOXIC?

When taken as a supplement, vitamin C can cause diarrhoea, nausea, burning urination or skin sensitivities. Reduce the dose if any of these should occur.

WATER-SOLUBLE VITAMINS

VITAMIN C IN THE DIET
SAMANTHA PARKER

For Samantha, aged 19, her first year at college was nearly her last. She fell behind in her work and failed her examinations because she had been off sick with so many colds and coughs.

When her doctor asked her what she ate each day, she replied:

'Coffee and a cigarette for breakfast, as I'm always on a diet and usually in a hurry. For lunch, I have a ham or cheese wholemeal sandwich, with an apple. In the evening I'm so tired that I have something quick like a bowl of cereal with skimmed milk, a boiled egg, or cheese on toast. Then I might go out for a drink with my friends, or if I'm studying I'll probably snack on popcorn or biscuits. At weekends I eat at work. I'm a waitress in a fast-food café so lunch is usually a burger. I do try to avoid the fries.'

Her doctor recommended that she should eat at least five servings of fresh fruit and vegetables each day, and take a vitamin C supplement when she had a cold or infection. He told her that even fries are a fairly good source of vitamin C, because they are cooked in oil, and we tend to eat large portions.

He also suggested that she should try to give up smoking. 'Every cigarette destroys 25mg of vitamin C,' he said. 'So you then have even less available to keep infections and tiredness at bay'.

Samantha took his advice, passed her re-sits and had no time off sick at all the following year. She even found enough energy to start playing tennis again.

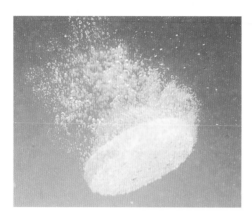

ABOVE *Avoid taking vitamin C at bedtime because it can act as a stimulant and keep you awake.*

WATER-
SOLUBLE
VITAMINS

Excess vitamin C is rapidly excreted in the urine, and it is unlikely that food sources alone will cause toxicity. Women who take the mini-pill (progesterone only) birth-control pill should not take more than 2g of vitamin C a day as this can reduce the effectiveness of the pill. You should consult your doctor about taking high-dose vitamin C supplements for long periods if you, or a close relation, have had kidney stones.

A GOOD COMBINATION

All minerals, particularly calcium and magnesium, and other vitamins help the body to make optimum use of vitamin C (see also vitamin P).

USING A SUPPLEMENT

Some nutritional experts believe that the basic requirement for adults is at least 500mg a day, but others disagree. Supplements are best taken in two or three doses. They are available as tablets, powders, liquid or effervescent preparations. Pure ascorbic acid can cause discomfort in the stomach and 'buffered' preparations are often better tolerated. Other formulations include sodium, calcium and magnesium ascorbate, and many contain vitamin P (see p39).

COOKING TIPS

You can minimize loss of vitamin C from food if you:

• Shop for fresh produce frequently, and buy it in good condition

• Store fruit and vegetables in a cool, dark place, preferably in a fridge

• Prepare produce just before eating, eat raw when possible or cook as briefly as possible

• Steam, stir-fry or use a microwave oven to cook vegetables. Avoid boiling, and never add bicarbonate of soda to the water

• Cook frozen vegetables without thawing first

• Do not soak fruit or vegetables, as the vitamin C drains away

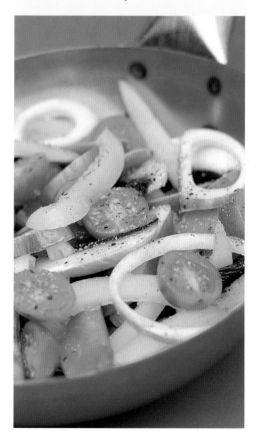

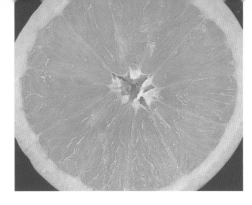

Vitamin P
bioflavonoids

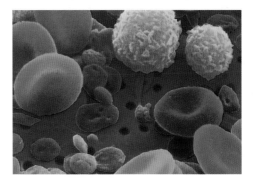

ABOVE *Red grapes are an excellent source of vitamin P and make a quick and tasty snack between meals.*

Vitamin P includes a number of substances that are normally found in the same foods as vitamin C. They are thought to aid the absorption of vitamin C and, possibly, to prolong its function. In addition, many of these substances are now known to be extremely active and, where they share similar functions, may even be more powerful than the better known vitamins C and E.

Vitamin P works with vitamin C to maintain the health of the thin walls of the small blood vessels known as capillaries, preventing bruising and bleeding, including excessive menstrual loss. Together, they also fight viruses and appear to reduce allergic conditions.

AVAILABILITY IN FOODS

Several hundred bioflavonoids have now been identified from a wide variety of foods, especially citrus fruits (where they are richest in the pith rather than the juice), red and blue berries and grapes, onions, garlic and buckwheat. Their absorption into the body may be slow and is sometimes incomplete, but they can be stored in small amounts. A diet rich in fruit and vegetables, especially those that are red, blue or purple in colour, can provide as much as one gram a day of these substances.

The bioflavonoids present in many foods appear to have slightly different actions. To make best use of their powerful anti-oxidant potential, eat as many different types as possible. Try drinking juices made from berries and grapes, especially black grapes, instead of tea and coffee. Consider taking some of the less palatable varieties, such as those from grape seeds, pine bark or ginko biloba, in the form of food supplements.

DEFICIENCY AND TOXICITY

Deficiency is unlikely if the diet contains fruit and vegetables, but if it does occur, it may result in bruising. There is no known toxicity.

USING A SUPPLEMENT

If you wish to take a supplement, vitamin P is best taken with vitamin C.

WATER-SOLUBLE VITAMINS

ABOVE *Vitamins C and P work together to strengthen the walls of the small blood vessels to prevent bruising and bleeding.*

Vitamin T

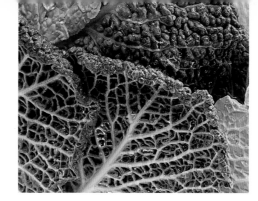

LEFT *Cabbage can be eaten raw, cooked or fermented (as sauerkraut).*

Little is known about vitamin T although it has been called the 'sesame seed factor'. It has also been found in egg yolks. It is thought to strengthen red blood cells. Toxicity is unknown and supplements are not available.

WATER-
SOLUBLE
VITAMINS

HOW DO I EAT SESAME SEEDS?

Sesame seed paste, also known as tahini, is sold in health-food shops. It can be used by itself as a spread or dip, or made into hummus by the addition of chickpeas (garbanzo beans) as in the recipe opposite. Hummus is now widely available in supermarkets.

(*Note. An increasing number of children are developing sesame seed allergies and in families prone to allergies, mothers may wish to avoid eating them in pregnancy or while breast feeding, or giving them to children under three.*)

Vitamin U

Vitamin U is found in raw cabbage. It is possible that it helps in healing ulcers of the skin and in the digestive tract. Toxicity is unknown and supplements are not available.

ABOVE *Sesame seeds can be made into a paste (tahini) or a sweet (halvah).*

HUMMUS

100g (4oz) canned chickpeas (garbanzo beans) (or cook your own from dried peas, in which case you can increase the nutritional value by sprouting them first – see p35).
1–2 crushed cloves of garlic according to your taste
1 tablespoon of olive oil
2 tablespoons of tahini (sesame seed paste)
juice of one lemon

METHOD
Whisk all the ingredients together in a liquidizer or food processor, until smooth. You may need to add a little water or vegetable stock.

Season with black or cayenne pepper or paprika.

Use as a dip with raw vegetables such as sticks of carrot, cauliflower florets, chicory, etc, or as a spread.

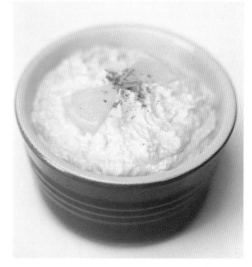

Vitamin A
retinol and beta-carotene

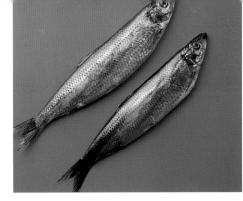

LEFT *Useful amounts of retinol are found in the flesh of oily fish such as herring.*

Vitamin A is essential for the health of the eyes. It prevents dry eye, a very common cause of blindness in the Third World, and improves eyesight, especially night vision. It boosts the immune system, helping to ward off infections, particularly those affecting the respiratory system and bladder. When taken with other anti-cancer nutrients, it is thought to reduce the risk of cancer. Vitamin A has an anti-oxidant function, which means that it neutralizes the unstable substances called free radicals that can cause damage, especially to the membranes of the cells.

LEFT *Cod liver oil and halibut liver oil are supplements that are naturally rich in vitamins A and D.*

Bones and teeth need vitamin A for healthy growth, and for repair after injury or surgery. The skin, which is constantly being replaced, requires vitamin A for the new cells to grow properly.

RIGHT *Whole milk products like cheese are a valuable source of retinol.*

FAT-SOLUBLE VITAMINS

AVAILABILITY IN FOODS

Vitamin A is fat-soluble and occurs as retinol in food from animal sources such as fish oil, liver, egg-yolk and whole-cream milk. The body can use it immediately or store it in the liver for future use. Retinol is destroyed by light, high temperatures, and when iron or copper utensils are used in cooking.

Beta-carotene and other carotenoids are sometimes called 'pro-vitamin A', as a proportion of them can, if needed, be converted into vitamin A in the intestine and liver.

They are present in yellow and orange vegetables and fruit. As they are water-soluble, they are lost from food if it is soaked in water for long periods. They are destroyed at high temperatures and by exposure to light.

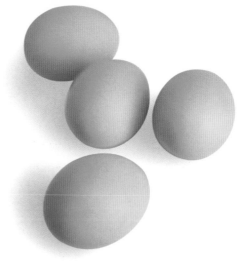

ABOVE *Eggs are relatively low in calories but rich in nutrients, including retinol.*

FAT-
SOLUBLE
VITAMINS

WHAT IF YOUR INTAKE IS TOO LOW?

Vitamin A is stored in the liver and symptoms of deficiency only occur when insufficient vitamin A is taken over a long period of time. Symptoms of deficiency include dry, itchy eyes that tire easily. Vision is poor in low light and adjusts slowly when going from light to dark. Severe deficiency can cause ulceration of the cornea and, eventually, blindness.

Infections, especially colds and sinus infections, may occur more frequently if your levels of vitamin A are low. The skin can become dry and bumpy, especially on the back of the arms, and infections such as acne or boils can develop. The hair becomes lustreless and the scalp dry and scurfy, especially if your diet is also deficient in protein.

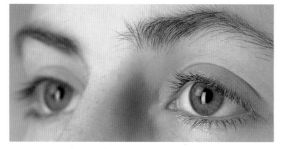

ABOVE *Without vitamin A the eyes become dry, and it can be difficult to see in poor light.*

If you take vitamin E in excess of about 180mcg daily, it may interfere with the absorption of beta-carotene.

WHEN EXTRA MAY BE NEEDED

• When the diet contains insufficient red and yellow fruit and vegetables, especially during rapid teenage growth, and in older people with small appetites
• If you regularly consume moderate or large amounts of alcohol
• If you eat a very low-fat diet, or a diet that is high in polyunsaturated fatty acids but low in vitamin E (see p47–50)
• If you are on a vegan diet
• If you have heavy or painful periods, or pre-menstrual syndrome
• If you smoke or live in a polluted area
• If you are stressed, especially from illness
• If you have diabetes or an under-active thyroid gland
• During pregnancy and when breast feeding
(*Pregnant and breast-feeding women should consult a doctor, midwife, or qualified nutritional therapist before taking any vitamin or mineral supplements.*)

ABOVE *The beta-carotene in leafy vegetables such as spinach can be converted into retinol in the body.*

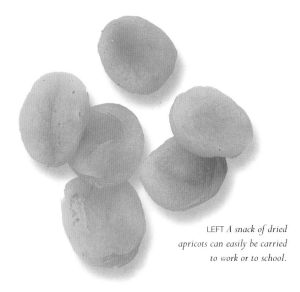

LEFT *A snack of dried apricots can easily be carried to work or to school.*

A GOOD COMBINATION

Vitamin A is most effective when protein, the B-vitamins, and vitamins C, D and E are present, as well as calcium, phosphorus and zinc. Zinc is also needed to release vitamin A stores.

VITAMIN A-RICH FRUIT SALAD

Choose fruits that you like, including those fruit rich in carotenoids such as apricots, bananas, cherries, mangoes, oranges, papayas, peaches, pineapple and raspberries. Out-of-season and tropical fruit, preferably preserved in juice rather than syrup, can be eaten from cans, as vitamin A is not lost in canning. Dried apricots and peaches can be soaked overnight.

METHOD

Allow about 200g (8oz) of fruit per person.
Chop into bite-sized pieces.
Cover with diluted orange juice (or juice from the tin if used) and chill.
Serve with cream or crème fraiche.

FAT-
SOLUBLE
VITAMINS

CAN TOO MUCH BE TOXIC?

Toxicity can occur with even relatively modest vitamin A supplementation when taken as retinol – for example, 15,000–30,000 mcg taken daily for longer than a month. Toxicity from food sources is unlikely unless liver, a particularly rich source of retinol, is eaten frequently.

However, despite its high iron content, liver should be avoided by pregnant women because even a single high dose of retinol can increase the risk of birth defects.

The symptoms of toxicity include pressure headaches, nausea and loss of appetite, abdominal pain, dizziness, irritability, menstrual problems, and skin changes which may manifest themselves as itchiness and dryness.

Pro-vitamin A from vegetable carotenoids does not cause toxicity, although an orange-yellow discoloration of the skin can develop if large amounts of carrot juice are drunk daily over a period of time. This discoloration of the skin will clear when the intake of vegetable carotenoids is reduced.

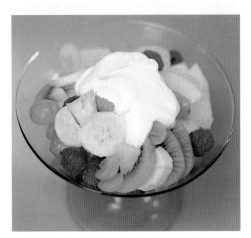

USING A SUPPLEMENT

If you wish to take a supplement of vitamin A, it is safest taken as beta-carotene.

DEALING WITH DEFICIENCY

The signs of vitamin A deficiency were first recognized by the Ancient Egyptians and dietary insufficiency remains a common problem throughout the world today. Even in developed countries it is thought that as many as 25 per cent of people do not eat enough of the foods that are rich in retinol and pro-vitamin A.

ABOVE
Cooked carrots provide more beta-carotene as it is released when the cell walls are damaged by heat.

In view of the potential toxicity of retinol, the pro-vitamin A found in fruit and vegetables is an important source of dietary vitamin A. (Beta-carotene can also be converted into vitamin A in the liver.) All adults should eat at least five servings of fruit and vegetables every day, because they are packed with minerals and fibre as well as vitamins and most of them contain no fat. To preserve all the nutrients, it is best to eat fruit and vegetables when they are fresh (i.e. in season) and, preferably, raw. If cooking is necessary, it should be done for as short a time as possible.

RIGHT *Spread taramasalata on wholemeal toast to make a nutritious starter or a quick and tasty snack.*

FAT-SOLUBLE VITAMINS

GOOD FOOD SOURCES OF VITAMIN A

Carotenoids – mcg per 100g (3½oz)

Carrots	12,000
Parsley	7,000
Spinach	6,000
Sweet potatoes	4,000
Pumpkin	3,000
Tomato purée	3,000
Apricots	2,000
Cantaloupes	2,000
Broccoli	2,000

(Note: *more than a hundred different carotenoids have been identified and these have individual amounts of vitamin A activity. Between 6 and 12mcg are equivalent to 1mcg of retinol.*)

Retinol – mcg per 100gm (3½oz)

Cooked calf's liver	40,000
Liver sausage	2,500
Butter	830
Fortified margarine	800
Cheddar cheese	320
Single cream	300
Cooked lamb's kidneys	100
Cooked herring	65
Taramasalata	40

(Note: *the dose of retinol in vitamin supplements is often given in International Units (IUs). To convert mcg to IUs, multiply by 3.33. For example, 100g of cheddar cheese contains 320x3.33=1,065IU.*)

Vitamin D
calciferol

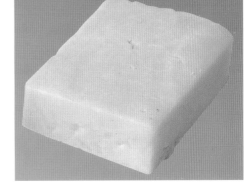

LEFT *Vitamin D and calcium in cheese add strength to bones and teeth.*

Vitamin D helps to maintain healthy bones and teeth and effective muscle function by regulating the levels of calcium and phosphorus in the body. In addition, it is needed to keep the heart and nervous system healthy, and to enable the blood to clot normally.

AVAILABILITY IN FOOD

Vitamin D is composed of several closely related substances that are present mainly in foods of animal origin, such as fatty fish, cod liver oil, eggs, milk, butter and cheese, but small amounts also occur in dark, green, leafy vegetables and mushrooms. It is sometimes known as the 'sunshine vitamin', as it can be manufactured in skin that is exposed to the sun without sunscreen. It is, therefore, a good idea to increase the amount taken in food during the winter. It can be stored in the body, so it is not essential to eat it every day.

RIGHT *Oily fish, such as mackerel, provide vitamin D.*

WHAT IF YOUR INTAKE IS TOO LOW?

Vitamin D deficiency in growing children causes rickets, a condition in which the muscles develop poorly and the bones are too soft. The weight-bearing bones of the legs bend, causing either bowed legs or knock-knees. In adults, loss of bone minerals from vitamin D deficiency causes osteomalacia, in which the bones are painful and tender, the muscles are weak and deafness develops. In older people, osteoporosis can occur when protein is lost from the bone in addition to the mineral loss. This is usually painless in its early stages (see also p61).

WHEN EXTRA MAY BE NEEDED

• If your skin is rarely exposed to sunlight (for example, night workers and those who regularly wear protective or all-enveloping clothing or uniform)
• By elderly people, especially in winter
• When you are pregnant or breast feeding
• If you live in an area where there is smog
• If you spend a large amount of time indoors
• If your skin is dark and you live in an area of little natural sunlight
• If you are a vegan
(Pregnant and breast-feeding women should consult a doctor, midwife, or qualified nutritional therapist before taking any vitamin or mineral supplements.)

FAT-SOLUBLE VITAMINS

CAN TOO MUCH BE TOXIC?

Too much vitamin D causes elevated levels of calcium in the blood, and results in drowsiness, nausea, weakness, excessive thirst, abdominal pain and a general feeling of malaise. Prolonged exposure to the sun can cause toxicity in white people whose skin is not already tanned (the dark outer skin shades the deeper layers of skin where the vitamin D is produced). In the longer term, calcium is deposited in the soft tissues of the body, including the walls of the blood vessels and the kidneys, where it can cause serious damage.

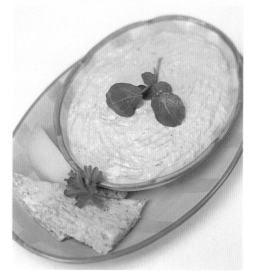

LEFT *Many breakfast cereals are fortified with vitamins, including vitamin D.*

A GOOD COMBINATION

Vitamin D is best utilized when vitamin A is also present. A balanced and adequate intake of calcium and phosphorus is also necessary.

USING A SUPPLEMENT

If you have sarcoidosis, do not take vitamin D supplements without consulting your doctor.

FAT-SOLUBLE VITAMINS

MACKEREL PATÉ

A quick recipe to top up the levels of vitamins D, F, C, many of the B-vitamins, and calcium.

SERVES 4
2 fillets of smoked mackerel
185g (6oz) cottage cheese
juice of half a lemon
salt and freshly milled pepper

METHOD
Place the ingredients in a liquidizer and blend until smooth.
  Serve chilled with buttered wholemeal bread and watercress or parsley to garnish.

GOOD FOOD SOURCES OF VITAMIN D

	mcg per 100g (3½oz)
Kippers	25
Mackerel	19
Tinned salmon	12.5
Tinned tuna	5
Cornflakes	2
Eggs	1.75

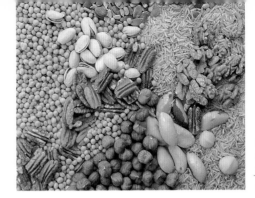

LEFT *Vegetable oils that are pressed from seeds are rich in vitamin E.*

Vitamin E
tocopherol

Vitamin E is a powerful anti-oxidant, which means that it neutralizes unstable substances known as free radicals that can cause damage, especially to the cell membranes. It is, therefore, able to provide protection against a wide variety of degenerative conditions, such as heart disease, strokes, senility, arthritis, diabetes and possibly cancer. It also helps to reduce the likelihood of blood clots forming in the blood vessels, causing blockage. Vitamin E promotes fertility, reduces or prevents the hot flushes of menopause, and protects the body from pollution. Stamina and endurance can be increased by adequate vitamin E intake.

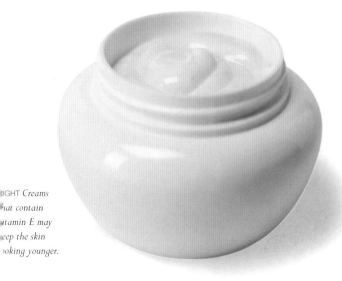

RIGHT *Creams that contain vitamin E may keep the skin looking younger.*

Vitamin E is particularly beneficial to the skin, both when taken in the diet and when vitamin E oil is applied externally to the skin. It helps to keep the skin looking younger, promotes healing and minimizes the risk of excessive scar formation. It has been reported to be beneficial for eczema, skin ulcers and viral infections, such as cold sores and shingles.

AVAILABILITY IN FOOD

Vitamin E is composed of a family of closely related substances that are present in vegetable oils, especially wheat germ oil, nuts, seeds, soy beans, whole grains, lettuce and other green vegetables. Vitamin E is easily lost in food processing, such as milling, cooking and freezing, and when food is stored or exposed to the air. Its qualities are preserved best if it is extracted from seeds and grains by cold pressing rather than by the use of heat or chemicals. It is less easily stored in the body than the other fat-soluble vitamins.

WHAT IF YOUR INTAKE IS TOO LOW?

Vitamin E deficiency is uncommon in healthy adults, and the symptoms are vague. They include fatigue, inflamed varicose veins, slow healing of wounds and burns, sub-fertility and premature ageing. Other symptoms, however, may be poorly identified and not specifically associated with vitamin E deficiency. Low levels

FAT-SOLUBLE VITAMINS

RIGHT
Vitamin E in nuts can be lost after shelling, when the kernel is exposed to the air.

of vitamin E in the blood have been found in association with a wide range of conditions such as acne, certain types of anaemia, gum disease, some types of gallstones and muscle disease, some kinds of dementia such as Alzheimer's disease, and some cancers.

WHEN EXTRA MAY BE NEEDED

- If you eat a lot of refined carbohydrates or fried food
- If your diet is high in polyunsaturated fats
- If you are prone to pre-menstrual symptoms, especially painful breasts, or have painful periods
- To reduce menopausal flushes and itching, especially of the vulva
- If you have poor circulation or suffer leg cramps at night
- If you have heart disease, or after a stroke
- If you suffer from Dupuytren's contracture (thickening of the ligaments of the hand)
- To relieve the painful or swollen joints caused by osteoarthritis
- When taking the birth-control pill or receiving hormone replacement therapy
- During pregnancy or when breast feeding
- If you are exposed to pollution, or drink chlorinated water

(Pregnant and breast-feeding women should consult a doctor, midwife, or qualified nutritional therapist before taking any vitamin or mineral supplements.)

GOOD FOOD SOURCES OF VITAMIN E

mg per 100g (3½oz)	
Wheat germ oil	190
Soya bean oil	87
Sunflower oil	27
Almonds	24.6
Walnuts	19.6
Cashew nuts (dry roasted)	11
Shrimps	6.6
Brown rice	2

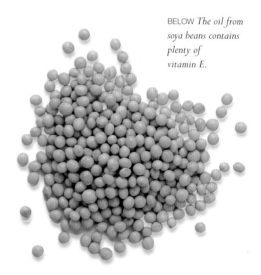

BELOW *The oil from soya beans contains plenty of vitamin E.*

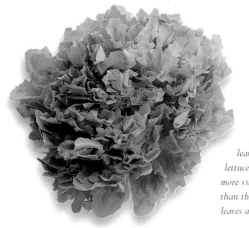

LEFT *The dark outer leaves of a lettuce contain more vitamin E than the paler leaves at its heart.*

CAN TOO MUCH BE TOXIC?

Toxicity is unlikely, as the body can eliminate any excess in the urine and faeces. A high intake of vitamin E can cause nausea, abdominal wind and diarrhoea. You should consult your doctor before taking supplements of vitamin E if you have high blood pressure, or take anti-coagulant ('blood thinning') medication or insulin.

A GOOD COMBINATION

Vitamin E is most effective when other anti-oxidant nutrients are present, including vitamin C, beta-carotene, and selenium. Other helpful nutrients are vitamin A, the B-vitamins, including inositol, and manganese.

USING A SUPPLEMENT

Vitamin E is destroyed by inorganic iron (ferrous sulphate), which should be taken at least eight hours apart from a vitamin E supplement. The other forms of iron are less likely to have this effect. Vitamin E supplements are less effective if taken at the same time as the birth-control pill. Vitamin E can also be absorbed through the skin, and this provides an alternative route for small amounts of vitamin E.

WAKE UP TO VITAMIN E

• Wheat germ is the isolated embryo of the wheat grain. It is crunchy, nutty and particularly rich in good nutrients. It is an excellent source of vitamin E, as well as the B-vitamins, selenium, zinc, phosphorus and magnesium. It is also a good source of dietary fibre, which helps to keep the bowel regular and protect against bowel cancer.

• Breakfast is often the easiest meal for introducing wheat germ which can be sprinkled onto any cereal. However, whole-grain cereals are the best as they also contain vitamin E and the B-vitamins. Be sure to buy wheat germ from a shop that has a good turnover so that it is as fresh as possible, and store it in the fridge.

FAT-SOLUBLE VITAMINS

BELOW *Wheat germ is the embryo removed from whole wheat.*

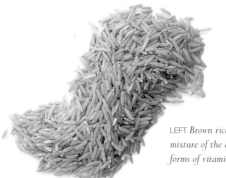

LEFT *Brown rice contains a mixture of the different forms of vitamin E.*

FAT-
SOLUBLE
VITAMINS

MAKING YOUR OWN MUESLI

Finding a brand of muesli to your own taste is not always easy, especially if you wish to avoid added sugar. Instead, buy a basic mix of your favourite grains, or make your own mix by buying the grains individually. Add sultanas and raisins, and keep in an airtight container. For variety, add different fruits and nuts each day, such as:

- Dried apricots, a banana and chopped almonds

- Grated apple and chopped hazel nuts

- Small cubes of pear and chopped walnuts

- Fresh raspberries or strawberries and chopped Brazil nuts

- Chopped dates, figs and banana chips or pecan nuts

Finally, sprinkle with wheat germ, and add yoghurt, milk or fruit juice. Sweeten with honey, dark brown sugar or even some molasses (see p26).

E IS FOR EVERYONE

The amount of vitamin E needed daily was originally estimated by measuring the amount that healthy people obtained in their diets, and assuming this to be adequate. However, many nutritionists believe that higher intakes of vitamin E may provide protection against chronic illnesses, including heart disease and possibly cancer.

We already know that vitamin E protects the body against the damaging effects of environmental pollution. This includes the chemicals in smog and cigarette smoke as well as dietary pollutants, such as the changes that occur when natural plant and fish oils are exposed to the oxygen in the air.

Vitamin E is also able to moderate the body's response to injury and to substances that cause allergic reactions. As a result, there is less pain and swelling after injury, and in allergic conditions such as hay fever, secretions from the eyes and nose may be reduced.

Vitamin E supplements can be taken to increase the daily intake of vitamin E but the mixture of different forms of vitamin E that occur naturally in food is likely to prove more effective than taking supplements.

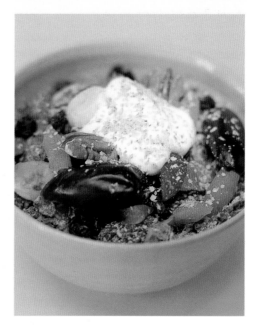

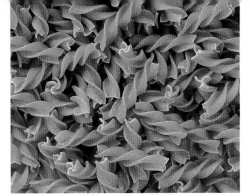

LEFT *Brown pasta contains more LA than white pasta.*

Vitamin F
essential fatty acids

Vitamin F is composed of two fatty acids: linoleic acid (LA) and alpha-linolenic acid (LNA). They are needed for normal growth and behaviour, healthy cell membranes, an effective immune system, and well-balanced hormone levels. They keep the skin and other tissues supple and youthful, and contribute towards the energy held in fat stores.

AVAILABILITY IN FOOD

LA and LNA are among the mix of fatty acids that make up the oils found in grains, nuts and seeds, but they are members of two distinct chemical families. Many nutritional experts believe that the large amount of refined food in the Western diet now means that many people do not get enough of the essential fatty acids, especially those in the LNA family. Ideally, the amount of LNA should be between one fifth to one half the amount of LA, which is more widely available in the modern diet.

LA and LNA are readily absorbed into the body, and can also be absorbed through the skin. They are not chemically stable when exposed to heat or air, and are easily lost during food processing.

WHAT IF YOUR INTAKE IS TOO LOW?

Excessive deficiency of LA can cause damage to the heart, kidneys and liver, and behavioural disturbance. Hair loss and eczema-like skin problems can occur, and there may be excessive

FAT-SOLUBLE VITAMINS

RIGHT *Oily fish, such as sardines, are an important source of vitamin F.*

sweating accompanied by thirst. The immune system may become less effective, causing slow healing and increased susceptibility to infection. Joints may become painful and stiff, and glands such as the tear and salivary glands can dry up.

In children, growth may be retarded; women may become more prone to miscarriage and men may be less fertile.

LNA deficiency can also cause growth retardation and skin dryness. Problems with vision,

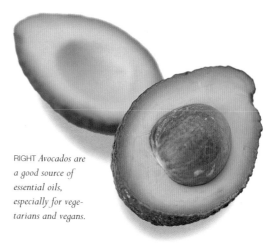

RIGHT *Avocados are a good source of essential oils, especially for vegetarians and vegans.*

OILS AND SLIMMING

• The low and very low-fat diets that are commonly advocated for slimming frequently ignore the fact that vitamin F is essential to health and, indeed, to life. Although foods that contain fats and oils are notoriously high in calories, only about one tablespoon of LA and two teaspoonfuls of LNA are needed each day, and this does not add up to a great number of calories.

• Good-quality oils are found in nuts, seeds and whole-grain cereals, such as brown rice and pasta, wholemeal bread, oatcakes, porridge and whole rye products. Two or three portions of oily fish (salmon, sardines, mackerel or tuna) should be eaten each week and you can treat yourself occasionally to avocados, which are also rich in good oils.

• The good news about the omega-3 oils is that they boost metabolism, increase energy and help the body to dump retained water. There have been reports of increased weight loss once flaxseed (linseed) oil was added to an already healthy diet. However, professional advice is needed if you wish to continue this supplement for longer than a few months.

learning, walking and behaviour can occur, and the arms and legs may develop a tingling sensation. The blood pressure and cholesterol levels may become elevated, and the blood may be more likely to clot, causing thrombosis.

WHEN EXTRA MAY BE NEEDED

• If you have dry skin, brittle nails or dandruff
• If you are overweight
• If you have pre-menstrual symptoms or benign breast lumps
• If you have dry eyes (Sjogren's syndrome) or cold hands and feet (Raynaud's disease)
• If you bruise easily
• If you have frequent infections
• If you are on a diet that is very low in fat
(Pregnant and breast-feeding women should consult a doctor, midwife, or qualified nutritional therapist before taking any vitamin or mineral supplements)

CAN TOO MUCH BE TOXIC?

Toxicity does not appear to be a problem for healthy people, but if you have any serious medical condition you should consult your doctor before starting to take supplements containing fatty acids.

A GOOD COMBINATION

A number of other nutrients are needed to ensure that LA, LNA and related fatty acids are able to function effectively. These include vitamins B3, B6, C, E and biotin, and the minerals zinc, magnesium and selenium.

USING A SUPPLEMENT

If you wish to take a supplement, commercial preparations containing a good balance between LA and LNA are now available. If your diet has been very low in LNA, flaxseed oil can be taken for a while, but imbalance between LA and LNA is likely after a few months. Always seek professional advice if you are in doubt.

LA and LNA should be obtained from a reputable source as the oils are not stable. It is important that light, air and heat are excluded from them during processing and storage. The bottles should be dark and carry a 'Use by' date.

RIGHT *Create a vitamin F feast with oatcakes and mackerel pâté (p46).*

INTRODUCING THE ESSENTIAL FATTY ACID FAMILIES

Rich food sources of LA	Rich food sources of LNA
Safflower seed	Flaxseed (linseed)
Sunflower seed	Hemp seed
Hemp seed	Canola (rapeseed)
Soybean	Soybean
Walnuts	Walnuts
Pumpkin seed	Dark green leaves
Sesame seed	
Flaxseed (linseed)	

A number of other oils and fats are closely related to LA and LNA and they can take over some, but not all, of the functions of LA and LNA when they are in short supply. Many of them are commercially available as food supplements and include:

Oils from the seeds of:	Some of the fats from:	Oils from cold water fish, such as:
Borage (starflower)	Meat and animal products	Salmon
Blackcurrant		Trout
Evening primrose		Mackerel
		Tuna

sold as Omega-3 fish oils

(Note: *These seed oils can aggravate epilepsy, and should be avoided if you have any form of epilepsy. If you have a blood disorder or bleeding problem, supplements of the fish oils should only be taken under medical supervision.*)

Vitamin K

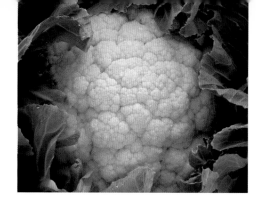

LEFT *As well as providing vitamin K, cauliflower appears to have cancer-inhibiting properties.*

Vitamin K is essential for normal clotting of the blood, and it helps in the formation of healthy bones and teeth.

AVAILABILITY IN FOODS

Vitamin K is present in leafy vegetables, cheese and liver. It is stable to heat, but can be destroyed by freezing and exposure to radiation and air pollution. Absorption can be decreased when rancid oils and fats, excessive sugar, aspirin, antibiotics, high doses of vitamin E or calcium, or mineral oils (for constipation) are taken at the same time. Little is stored in the body, but it can be made in the intestine where its production is enhanced by cultured milk products, such as yoghurt.

BELOW *Nutritious raw tomatoes can be used in a wide selection of meals and salads to suit all tastes.*

WHAT IF YOUR INTAKE IS TOO LOW?

Insufficient vitamin K can cause nosebleeds, internal haemorrhage or miscarriage, but these complaints are rare unless other medical conditions are also present.

WHEN EXTRA MAY BE NEEDED

• If you have heavy periods or bruise easily
• During pregnancy
(Pregnant and breast-feeding women should consult a doctor, midwife, or qualified nutritional therapist before taking any vitamin or mineral supplements.)

CAN TOO MUCH BE TOXIC?

Toxicity is unlikely when vitamin K is obtained from food or alfalfa tablets (see p98), but can occur with the synthetic compound vitamin K3, or menadione. Symptoms of toxicity include

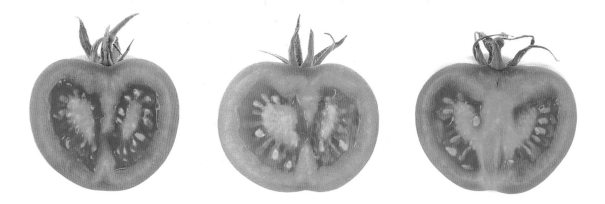

flushing, sweating or a feeling of chest constriction. Anaemia may also occur.

A GOOD COMBINATION

None has yet been recognized.

USING A SUPPLEMENT

If you take anti-coagulant medicines (to prevent blood clots), consult your doctor before taking a supplement of vitamin K.

LEFT *By eating your broccoli fresh rather than freezing it first, you will gain the most benefit from its high vitamin K content.*

GOOD FOOD SOURCES OF VITAMIN K

mcg per 100g (3½oz)

Cauliflower	3,600
Brussels sprouts	800
Broccoli	800
Lettuce	700
Spinach	600
Pig's liver	600
Tomatoes	400
Cabbage	400
String beans	290
Lean meat	100

FAT-SOLUBLE VITAMINS

VITAMIN K AND THE NEW BORN

Vitamin K was discovered in Germany in 1929, and the designation 'K' was taken from the word 'koagulation'. The absence of vitamin K was found to be the reason why the blood of chicks failed to coagulate normally when they were fed on a fat-free diet.

Vitamin K deficiency is rare but since the vitamin does not pass through the placenta, newly born infants have low reserves. They are unable to make their own vitamin K because they do not have any bacteria in their intestines and, without vitamin K, their blood will not clot normally for about four days after birth.

If there is a risk of bleeding into a baby's brain, for example, after a complicated labour or forceps delivery, doctors often administer vitamin K after birth. At one time it was always given by injection, but some doctors believe that this way of administering vitamin K might increase the risk of the child developing leukaemia later in life. Although this link has not been proved, vitamin K is now usually administered by mouth.

In certain countries, vitamin K is routinely given to new-born babies as it is very difficult to be sure that no minor injury has occurred during the birth. Parents who would prefer vitamin K not to be given to their babies should discuss this with the obstetrician before the mother goes into labour.

In cultures that practise the circumcision of baby boys, this operation is usually postponed until a few days after birth of the baby to avoid the risk of haemorrhage.

Getting to know your minerals

Minerals are incorporated into the structure of the body and the body needs a regular supply of many minerals in greater quantities than vitamins. Those minerals that are needed in amounts greater than 100mg per day are sometimes called macrominerals. These include calcium, magnesium, phosphorus, sodium, potassium, sulphur and chlorine. The other minerals needed by the body are usually referred to as trace minerals. It is likely that the list of trace minerals that are essential to health will grow longer as the ability to measure very small amounts of minerals improves.

MINERALS

As yet, only a limited number of minerals have been included in the official lists that provide recommendations for daily intake (see p130–139). Despite this, mineral deficiencies are probably more common than vitamin deficiencies, especially in people whose calorie intake is limited for any reason, and in women whose needs are increased during pregnancy and when breast feeding.

A sufficient intake of minerals is best achieved by eating a wide range of different whole foods, preferably organically grown, and avoiding high-calorie foods, as well as white flour and sugar, from which the rich natural mineral content has been removed during food processing. It is also wise to avoid excessive caffeine and alcohol, which can deplete the body of minerals. This approach allows the body to exercise its own finely tuned mechanisms for selecting and absorbing the minerals that it needs to top up its stores.

Taking mineral supplements can be tricky, as minerals compete with each other for absorption into the body across the wall of the intestine. For example, large amounts of calcium can reduce absorption of magnesium, phosphorus, zinc and manganese, and excessive zinc can reduce the absorption of copper, iron and phosphorus. Phosphorus is probably already too plentiful in the diet of many people in developed countries, and an excess of this mineral can block the absorption of many other minerals.

If you wish to take mineral supplements, it is probably best to choose preparations that contain a balanced selection of minerals. If you feel that you need to supplement individual minerals in addition to this, it would be wise to seek professional advice before doing so.

Calcium, magnesium and phosphorus

LEFT *Eat the bones of the sardines as well. It may sound unappealing but they are a good source of calcium.*

With the growing concern about osteoporosis, much attention has been paid to ensuring there is enough calcium in the diet. Many nutritionists are also concerned that the average diet in developed countries does not supply enough magnesium and contains excessive phosphorus. The balance between these three minerals in the body is critical for healthy bones, but they are both work mates and rivals. Acting together, they build up the bones in early life and maintain the skeleton later on in life. They also work together to relay messages along the nerves, and to enable muscles to function normally. Unfortunately, they compete with one another for absorption into the body, and phosphorus is more easily absorbed than the other two. When the diet is unbalanced, one way for the body to restore the correct proportions is to sacrifice some of the calcium that is stored in the bones.

Calcium is the most abundant mineral in the body, weighing in at about 1.5kg (3lb) for each adult. It stabilizes many body functions, has an important role in blood clotting, and almost certainly helps to prevent bowel cancer. Calcium is a natural tranquillizer, so a milky drink at night will help you to sleep well.

Magnesium is essential for all the major processes of the body. The small amount present in the body helps to release energy from food, to build new cells and proteins, and has a major role in enabling muscles to relax, including those in the walls of arteries, where it may help to prevent raised blood pressure.

Phosphorus is the second most abundant mineral in the body. It is vital for the production of energy and is an essential component of cell membranes. It also enables a number of B-vitamins to function effectively.

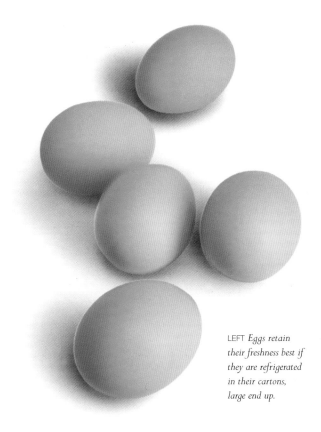

LEFT *Eggs retain their freshness best if they are refrigerated in their cartons, large end up.*

MINERALS

AVAILABILITY IN FOOD

Even when dietary supplies of calcium and magnesium are adequate, neither mineral is easily absorbed from the intestine. Diets that are high in protein, fat or phosphorus can lead to deficiency, as can a sedentary lifestyle. Absorption is also reduced if the stomach secretes insufficient acid, for example in the elderly, after surgery or in pernicious anaemia.

Calcium is widely available in food, but few foods contain it in large amounts. The richest sources include milk and milk products, beans, nuts, molasses and fruits. It cannot be absorbed unless vitamin D is also available either in the diet or from the action of the sun on the skin.

Magnesium can be found in vegetables, but the amount they contain depends on the amount of magnesium in the soil. In recent years, magnesium has been lost from the soil through acid rain and the application of chemical fertilizers. It is present in most nuts, seeds and whole

LEFT *Nuts provide plenty of magnesium and make a quick and easy snack.*

grains, but up to 85 per cent can be lost from whole grains when they are milled.

When foods are boiled, magnesium leaches into the water; this can be retrieved if you use the water in gravy or soup. Phosphorus is available in meats, poultry, eggs and seeds. Colas and other fizzy drinks are high in phosphorus, and drinking large quantities can make a significant contribution to the excessive intake that concerns some nutritionists.

WHAT IF YOUR INTAKE IS TOO LOW?

Excessive, long-term calcium deficiency causes rickets, osteomalacia (see vitamin D, p45) and osteoporosis. It may increase the risk of tooth decay, gum disease, deafness, toxaemia of pregnancy, muscle aches and cramps, anxiety, painful and heavy periods, cataracts and, in children, impaired growth and behavioural problems.

Magnesium deficiency causes fatigue, loss of appetite, insomnia, apathy and poor memory. Lack of magnesium can cause painful periods in women and spasm of the muscles in the walls of the arteries, which may raise blood pressure. It may also contribute to incontinence in the elderly and bed-wetting in children.

Phosphorus deficiency is very uncommon, but symptoms of severe deficiency include

BELOW *Seeds are a rich and valuable source of calcium if you do not drink milk or eat many dairy produce.*

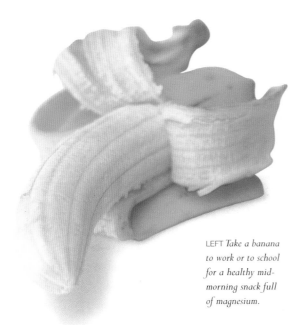

LEFT *Take a banana to work or to school for a healthy mid-morning snack full of magnesium.*

muscle weakness, loss of appetite, increased susceptibility to infection, anaemia and, in children, poor growth and rickets.

WHEN EXTRA CALCIUM AND MAGNESIUM MAY BE NEEDED

• If you live in a soft-water area or drink bottled water that has a low mineral content
• If your diet consists mostly of processed foods, or contains excessive protein, fat, sugar, caffeine, salt or fizzy drinks
• If you regularly consume moderate or large amounts of alcohol
• If you have heavy or painful periods, or are prone to pre-menstrual symptoms
• If you are at risk of osteoporosis (take only under medical supervision)
• During pregnancy and when breast feeding
• When taking the birth-control pill regularly, diuretics (water pills), antacid preparations (for indigestion) or receiving hormone replacement therapy

---

WHEN EXTRA CALCIUM MAY BE NEEDED

• When you are lacking in vitamin D (see p45)
• If you have gum disease, such as gingivitis

WHEN EXTRA MAGNESIUM MAY BE NEEDED

• If losses of magnesium from the body are high: such as in urine when taking diuretics (water tablets), in faeces if you have diarrhoea or pass loose stools, or in sweat if you perspire excessively from heat or exercise
• If you regularly take large amounts of vitamin C daily (more than 1,000mg)

WHEN EXTRA PHOSPHORUS MAY BE NEEDED

• If you regularly consume moderate or large amounts of alcohol
• If you are taking antacid preparations for indigestion or stomach ulcers
• During pregnancy
• If you have osteo-porosis (take only under medical supervision)

MINERALS

RIGHT *Keep your bones strong by replacing caffeine drinks with fruit juice which is rich in minerals.*

(Pregnant and breast-feeding women should consult a doctor, midwife, or qualified nutritionist before taking any mineral or vitamin supplement.)

CAN TOO MUCH BE TOXIC?

Calcium excess is easily eliminated in the short term in the urine and faeces. If excess calcium is combined with magnesium deficiency, calcium can be deposited in the soft tissues, including the kidneys, and cause damage. In the long term, excessive calcium may cause kidney stones, weakness, constipation, abdominal pain, decreased appetite and nausea. There is some concern that

LEFT *Bones are strengthened when they are stressed, for example, during weight-bearing exercise.*

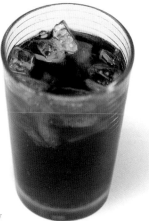

RIGHT *Too many fizzy drinks which have a high phosphorus content may cause calcium loss through the kidneys.*

excessive calcium may contribute to atherosclerosis (hardening of the arteries), eventually causing dementia. Further research is needed, but it may be wise to avoid high doses of calcium over a long period of time, unless there is a good medical reason.

Magnesium overload is virtually unknown because any excess is rapidly eliminated from the kidneys and in the faeces. However, toxicity can occur if calcium levels are low, especially if magnesium supplements are given by injection. Symptoms include muscle weakness and fatigue.

Phosphorus is not toxic on its own. However, excessive phosphorus can contribute to the symptoms of calcium deficiency, including osteoporosis. When there is too little calcium relative to phosphorus, there are increased risks of high blood pressure and bowel cancer.

A GOOD COMBINATION

Nutritionists suggest that a balanced diet should provide one to two parts each of calcium and phosphorus to one part of magnesium. Calcium is best absorbed in the presence of vitamin A and vitamin D as well as iron, and it is found to be most effective in the body when vitamin D, unsaturated fats, and manganese are present.

Magnesium is most effective in the presence of vitamins B6, C, D, and protein.

Phosphorus requires vitamins A and D, iron, manganese, adequate protein and unsaturated fatty acids to be most effective.

USING A SUPPLEMENT

Calcium and magnesium should normally be taken together and the amount absorbed depends on the form in which they are taken. Dolomite and bonemeal contain both minerals and appear to be fairly well absorbed, but there have been concerns about contamination from lead and other toxic metals and it is best to choose a preparation that is specified as being contaminant-free.

Of the chemical preparations, calcium is probably absorbed best when taken as the aspartate or citrate salts, and magnesium as the gluconate salt, or when chelated with amino acids. Magnesium oxide and sulphate are also useful preparations.

MINERALS

BUILDING AND MAINTAINING GOOD BONES

In osteoporosis, the bones lose both minerals and protein and as we get older, this increases the risk of fracture. Although osteoporosis is more common in women, it is now being diagnosed with increasing frequency in men.

It is far better to prevent osteoporosis than to try to treat or cure it, and this means building up strong bones in the first 30 years of life. However, it is never too late to pay proper attention to your bones and recent research shows that even in later years the condition can be slowed down or even reversed.

How is this done?

You can strengthen your bones if you take the following measures:

• Eat a diet that contains plenty of calcium, but make sure that it is balanced with a good supply of magnesium. Other helpful nutrients are boron, manganese, copper and vitamin K.

• Make sure that you obtain enough vitamin D in your diet and by exposing your skin to the sun, without sunscreen lotion, for 10 minutes before 10 am or in the late afternoon. Never expose unprotected skin for any longer.

You can also minimize the loss of calcium from the bones by:

• Avoiding too much protein in the diet: this helps to prevent a high phosphorus intake

• Cutting down on caffeine (in tea, coffee, and many over-the-counter painkillers), salt and alcohol

• Giving up smoking.

• Taking exercise for 30 minutes at least three times a week. Walking will help to protect the bones in your legs and spine. Tennis, rowing, gardening or simple weight training will strengthen the upper body.

• Avoiding laxatives and antacids that contain aluminium (if they are needed, use those that contain calcium).

• Not reducing your weight to below that recommended for your height.

• Women may wish to consider hormone replacement therapy in consultation with their doctor.

ABOVE *When you eat a milk product, try to include a magnesium-rich food as well.*

As the body's absorption of calcium and magnesium can be altered by food, supplements with a little vitamin C may be most efficiently taken between meals or at bedtime, when they may also enhance sleep. Preparations that include hydrochloric acid and vitamin D are well absorbed by the body.

Phosphorus supplements are rarely needed and would require extra calcium and magnesium. Small amounts are contained in some multi-mineral preparations, but you should seek medical advice if you wish to take higher doses.

BANISH PAINFUL PERIODS

Extra magnesium can help relieve painful periods, and ideally this should come from a well-balanced diet. If a supplement is needed, it may be advisable to take equal amounts of magnesium and calcium for a short time. Vitamins E and B6 plus a general multi-mineral and vitamin preparation can also help.

SARDINE PATÉ

This pâté can be easily prepared in minutes and is rich in both calcium and magnesium. The amount of phosphorus is rather high, but the balance would be improved if a tomato (see Boron, p64), a banana and a glass of orange juice were added to complete a light meal.

SERVES FOUR

200g (7oz) tinned sardines with bones, drained
100g (4oz) curd cheese
2-3 tablespoons of lemon juice
2 tablespoons of single cream
salt and pepper
wholemeal toast and lemon wedges to serve

METHOD

Place the first four ingredients in a liquidizer. Blend briefly and season to taste.

Serve with wholemeal toast and garnish with lemon wedges.

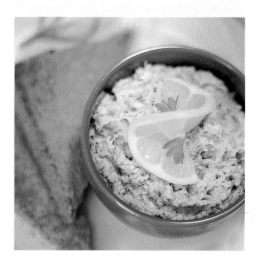

THE CALCIUM, MAGNESIUM AND PHOSPHORUS
CONTENT OF SOME COMMON FOODS

	Calcium mg per 100g (3½oz)	Magnesium mg per 100g (3½oz)	Phosphorus mg per 100g (3½oz)
Cheddar cheese*	800	25	520
Spinach	600	59	93
Sardines	368	36	472
Brewer's yeast	210	231	1,753
Brazil nuts	180	410	590
Yoghurt*	170	18	140
Blackstrap molasses	685	258	85
Sunflower seeds	120	39	837
Whole milk*	120	12	95
Haricot beans, boiled	65	45	120
Chick peas (garbanzo beans), cooked	64	67	130
Walnuts	61	130	510
Shrimps	60	36	206
Winter cabbage, raw	57	17	54
Eggs, boiled	52	12	220
Hazel nuts	44	56	230
Flour, wholemeal	35	140	340
Flour, white non-fortified	15	36	130
Apricots, stewed	34	24	44
Lettuce	23	8	27
Broad beans, cooked	21	28	99
Avocado	15	29	31
Orange juice	12	12	22
Chicken, cooked	11	24	190
Banana	7	42	28

MINERALS

* Milk is well known to be rich in calcium, but it is relatively poor in magnesium. You should, therefore, try to avoid depending too heavily on milk or milk products for calcium. Seeds, nuts, pulses and dark green leafy vegetables all provide a better proportion of magnesium.

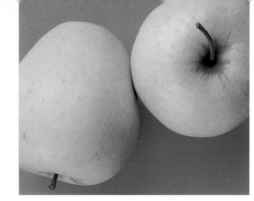

LEFT *Apples can help to strengthen your bones and also support your immune system.*

FAR LEFT *Grapes are rich in minerals including boron.*

Boron

Boron is now thought to help prevent osteoporosis by reducing the loss of calcium and magnesium in the urine. It may also alleviate menopausal symptoms in women, by increasing the level of oestradiol, a particularly active type of oestrogen. It may also reduce the symptoms of arthritis.

MINERALS

AVAILABILITY IN FOODS

The best sources of boron are fresh fruits, such as apples, pears and grapes, and dried fruits such as apricots and prunes. It is also found in leafy green vegetables, members of the bean family and nuts.

WHAT IF YOUR INTAKE IS TOO LOW?

Insufficient boron may adversely affect the calcium, magnesium and phosphorus balance in the body (see p57) and cause thinning of the bones, as well as increasing the risks of high blood pressure and arthritis.

WHEN EXTRA MAY BE NEEDED

If you eat mainly refined foods and insufficient fruit. *(Pregnant and breast-feeding women should consult a doctor, midwife, or qualified nutritionist before taking any mineral or vitamin supplement.)*

CAN TOO MUCH BE TOXIC?

Until recently, boron was used medically only for external application, for example, on the skin as an antiseptic in the form of boric acid. Ingestion of preparations containing boron caused dryness of the skin and problems with the digestive system. However, boron as a supplement, which is taken at a much lower dose, has shown no evidence of toxicity as yet.

A GOOD COMBINATION

Boron is most effective when supplies of manganese, calcium and vitamin B2 are also present in the body.

USING A SUPPLEMENT

A number of manufacturers now include amounts of boron in commercial preparations which have been designed to alleviate menopausal symptoms or to help maintain strong, healthy bones.

GOOD FOOD SOURCES OF BORON

mg per 100g (3½oz)	
Tomatoes	12
Pears	10
Apples	7
Prunes	3

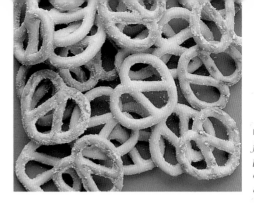

LEFT *Manufactured foods, such as pretzels, often contain large amounts of salt.*

Potassium and sodium

Among the constituents of the blood that doctors measure most frequently are the levels of potassium, sodium and chloride. The balance between these 'electrolytes', as they are known, is vital. Together they regulate the amount of water in the body and the delicate balance of where it is distributed. The highest level of potassium is found inside the cells. Sodium is mainly in the fluid around the cells and also surrounding the cells of the blood. However, it is the manner in which sodium and potassium are exchanged across the cell membranes that enables the nervous system to transmit messages and the muscles to contract and relax.

RIGHT
*f your diet
ontains a lot of
alt, you may need
o balance it with
extra potassium.*

Potassium is the mineral that is most commonly supplemented by doctors. This is usually to replace the potassium lost in the urine as a result of taking diuretic (water) tablets. Potassium is essential for normal growth and for building muscle.

Sodium chloride (salt) is needed for the production of hydrochloric acid in the stomach. This aids digestion and helps to protect the body against any infectious organisms present in food.

AVAILABILITY IN FOODS

Potassium is present in fruit and vegetables, as well as in whole grains, fish and unprocessed meat. It is lost from food during the canning process. About 90 per cent of the potassium in the diet is absorbed, but it is not stored in the body.

Sodium is 100 per cent absorbed from food, but only about 10 per cent of that present in the average Western diet is actually needed. Fortunately, it is easily lost in the urine, but in case of sudden need, a little is stored in the bones. Most natural foods contain little sodium, but it is added in food preparation as salt, which is the common name for sodium chloride.

MINERALS

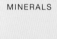

LEFT *Olives are naturally low in sodium unless they are preserved in brine.*

Other sources include water-softening units that use sodium, baking powder and the flavour enhancer monosodium glutamate.

WHAT IF YOUR INTAKE IS TOO LOW?

Potassium deficiency initially causes fatigue, muscle weakness, slow reflexes and dry skin or acne. Mood changes, such as depression, can develop with further deficiency, and the heart may start to beat irregularly. A severe deficit can cause raised blood sugar, bone thinning, a very slow heart rate and even death.

Deficiency is rare, as sodium is so plentiful in the diet in developed countries. However, deficiency can occur when sodium is lost in body fluids, such as in diarrhoea and vomiting, or excessive sweating. Symptoms of sodium deficiency include nausea, dizziness, poor concentration and memory, drowsiness and

LEFT *Dried fruit contains plenty of potassium and can be an alternative to salty snacks.*

LEFT *Restrict your cheese intake if you are on a low-salt diet.*

muscle weakness. If the deficiency is untreated, the blood pressure can drop catastrophically.

WHEN EXTRA POTASSIUM AND SODIUM MAY BE NEEDED

- After excessive sweating (e.g. through exercise)
- If you have diarrhoea and/or vomiting

WHEN EXTRA POTASSIUM MAY BE NEEDED

- If your diet contains excessive amounts of processed foods, which often contain salt or sugar
- If you regularly consume large amounts of coffee or other caffeine drinks, or alcohol
- If you take diuretic (water) tablets (check with your doctor first, as some of these tablets can conserve potassium)
- If you regularly take laxatives

(Pregnant and breast-feeding women should consult a doctor, midwife, or qualified nutritionist before taking any mineral or vitamin supplement.)

CAN TOO MUCH BE TOXIC?

Potassium can be toxic in excess, and this affects heart function. However, toxicity usually occurs only during illness, such as kidney failure.

Sodium in excess can cause high blood pressure in those people who are particularly sensitive to sodium (see Easing your heart's load, p68).

A GOOD COMBINATION

Many nutritionists recommend an intake of twice as much potassium as sodium. Potassium has been shown to be most effective in the presence of vitamin B6, and sodium acts best when vitamin D is present.

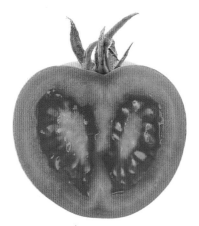

ABOVE *Feast on potassium with a tomato and basil salad — a perfect accompaniment to Mediterranean meals.*

GOOD FOOD SOURCES OF POTASSIUM

mg per 100g (3½oz)

Instant coffee	4,000
Dried fruit	700–1,800
Molasses	1,500
Raw salad vegetables	150–1,000
French fries	1,000
Nuts	400–900
Salmon	470
Banana	350
Raw broccoli	340
Raw tomatoes	290
Raw white cabbage	280
Lamb	240
Melon	220–320
Raspberries	220
Oranges	180

FOODS THAT CONTAIN A HIGH PROPORTION OF SODIUM

mg per 100g (3½oz)

Yeast extract	4,600
Olives in brine	2,250
Bacon	1,900
Smoked fish	1,000–1,800
Salami	1,800
Pretzels	1,600
Cornflakes	1,200
Stilton cheese	1,150
Corned beef	910
Salted butter	870
Margarine	800
Sausages	780
Sauerkraut	750
Bread	560

(Food labels and sodium: the label usually states salt content, and you may well find different levels from those quoted above. Divide the salt content by 2.5 to calculate the sodium content. For example, 5g of salt (about a teaspoonful) contains 2g sodium.)

MINERALS

USING A SUPPLEMENT

Anyone who eats the recommended five portions (each portion approximately 100g or 3½oz) of fruit and vegetables every day is unlikely to be deficient in potassium. 'Low sodium' table salt contains potassium chloride, and provides an easy way to increase your intake of potassium while, at the same time, limiting your sodium intake. Labels on over-the-counter potassium supplements often give the content in milli-equivalents: 1meq=64mg.

Sodium supplements are only needed when there are fluid losses from the body (see Active living p122–123).

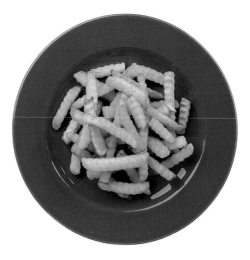

ABOVE *If you like lots of salt with your fries, use low sodium table salt to boost your potassium intake.*

DID YOU KNOW?

Even one single serving of fresh fruit or vegetables every day appears to reduce by around 40 per cent the chance that you will have a stroke. The potassium, magnesium and fibre that is found in fruit and vegetables work together to control blood pressure.

EASING YOUR HEART'S LOAD

If you have high blood pressure, it is a sign that your heart is working harder. This can lead to heart failure or a heart attack, and also increases the risk of a stroke.

Many people limit the amount of salt in their diets in the hope that this will either prevent high blood pressure, or at least help to reduce the likelihood that it will occur. With the exception of a few people, who do seem to have a particular sensitivity to salt, there is little scientific evidence to support this action.

Research suggests that a diet containing ample potassium may provide more protection against high blood pressure than a diet that is low in sodium. Vegetarians and people who live in more primitive cultures, where very little salt is eaten, are less likely to have high blood pressure. Both these groups eat large amounts of fruit and vegetables, which provide very good supplies of potassium.

This does not mean that a diet that is high in salt is advisable: you do not need much salt and you may be someone whose blood pressure is sensitive to salt.

If you reduce your salt intake gradually, you may find your taste for it changes, and you may no longer need to add extra salt. Try using more herbs and spices to flavour your food instead.

PACK IN THE POTASSIUM

Chilled, freshly prepared fruit drinks can help to get you going in the morning and pick you up when you are tired. They top up your potassium levels for the day, and take just a few minutes to prepare.

SUGGESTED COMBINATIONS

• 1 banana and two peeled oranges (or use 280 ml (10 fl. oz) fresh orange juice)
• 2 eating apples, cored but not peeled and 120g (4oz) of your favourite berries, fresh or frozen
• 200g (7oz) fresh pineapple or pineapple juice and two pears, cored but not peeled
• 6-8 fresh stoned fruit, e.g. peaches, nectarines or plums, and 4 fresh dates (but remove stones first)

METHOD

Choose one of the fruit combinations suggested, or create your own.

Combine ingredients together in a liquidizer. Add spring water (sparkling or flat), from the fridge, and/or ice cubes to create the consistency you prefer.

Flavour with your favourite spices, such as cinnamon, if desired.

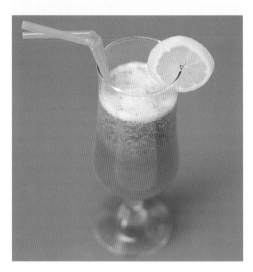

Toxic minerals

Since the start of industrial processes, people have been exposed to toxic minerals, but certain nutrients can enable the body to deal with low-level exposure.

CADMIUM

Sources of cadmium include cigarettes, nickel-cadmium batteries, phosphate fertilizers and the water from corroded pipes. Cadmium poisoning can contribute to high blood pressure, hardening of the arteries, heart attacks, strokes, bone pain and enlargement of the prostate gland.

Nutritional protection is provided by a diet that contains plenty of zinc and vitamin C.

LEAD

Car exhausts, industrial emissions, many industrial processes, and cigarette smoking are major sources of lead, as was leaded paint. It is assimilated into the body more easily when inhaled than when it is taken by mouth. Lead poisoning causes mood changes, mental retardation, hyperactivity in children, diminished fertility, high blood pressure and death. It is best to avoid exposure to lead, but certain nutrients, including calcium, and vitamins A and C, also help to reduce its effects.

MERCURY

Mercury or 'quicksilver' is a major industrial pollutant that today may contaminate lakes and seas and the fish that live in them. It is also present in insecticides, anti-fungal dressings for seeds, and dental amalgam. Symptoms of toxicity include fatigue, sleep disturbance, irritability, loss of libido and serious damage to the nervous system. Protective nutrients include selenium, vitamins A, C, and E, and the B-vitamins.

MINERALS

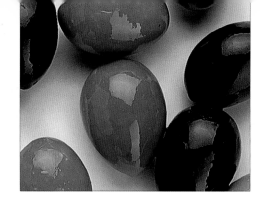

LEFT *Olives preserved in brine are a good source of chlorine, but are high in sodium.*

Chloride

MINERALS

Chloride is formed when the gas chlorine is dissolved in water. It works with potassium and sodium to control the passage of fluid in the blood vessels and the tissues, and to regulate acidity in the body. It is also an important part of hydrochloric acid, secreted by the stomach to digest food.

AVAILABILITY IN FOODS

For most people a major source of chloride is table salt, but it is also present in vegetable seaweed, such as dulse and kelp, as well as in olives, rye, watercress, tomatoes and celery. It is widely used in the water purification industry, but this evaporates, as chlorine, from tap water when it is boiled.

WHAT IF YOUR INTAKE IS TOO LOW?

Deficiency may cause the loss of too much potassium in the urine, resulting in weakness, and a drop in blood pressure.

WHEN EXTRA MAY BE NEEDED

If your losses are greater than your intake, for example, when you sweat excessively, or if you have diarrhoea, or are vomiting.

CAN TOO MUCH BE TOXIC?

Fluid retention may occur, but this is mostly as a result of too much sodium.

A GOOD COMBINATION

No information is currently available.

USING A SUPPLEMENT

Deficiency is extremely unlikely to occur in healthy adults.

LEFT *Add celery to salads and vegetable dishes or eat it raw as a crudité or with peanut butter.*

GOOD FOOD SOURCES OF CHLORINE

mg per 100g (3½oz)	
Common salt	6,100
Potassium chloride (used in salt substitutes)	4,800
Olives in brine	3,750
Tomato juice	370
Raw celery	180
Watercress	160
Baked potato with skin	94
Lettuce	53

Iron

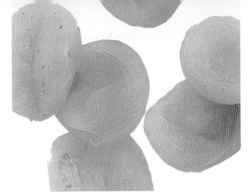

Iron is needed for the manufacture of red blood cells. Deficiency is common and causes a particular type of anaemia. This often occurs in women of childbearing age, who need extra iron to replace that lost in their monthly periods, and also during pregnancy, when iron is needed by the baby. Others at risk of insufficient iron in the diet include bottle-fed babies, as the iron in formula milk is less readily absorbed than that in breast milk, and toddlers and adolescents who are growing rapidly and often do not eat enough food containing iron. Poor absorption of iron can occur in the elderly.

RIGHT
Seeds are a good source of iron for vegetarians, vegans or anyone who doesn't eat much meat.

deficient, but they do need to think more carefully about their diet than meat eaters.

Absorption of iron can be reduced by the oxalic acid found in spinach and Swiss chard and by certain substances found in grains, soy and other pulses, tea and coffee. Ideally, tea and coffee should be avoided at mealtimes.

WHAT IF YOUR INTAKE IS TOO LOW?

Iron deficiency can cause anaemia. Symptoms of anaemia include fatigue, poor stamina, palpitations of the heart and shortness of breath after very little exertion, a sore tongue and cracks at the corners of the mouth, problems with swallowing, and changes in the fingernails which become concave and 'spoon shaped'. Children may develop learning difficulties, grow slowly and occasionally start to eat earth and other abnormal substances; a condition that is known as 'pica'.

MINERALS

AVAILABILITY IN FOODS

Red meats are good sources of iron, because the iron they contain is in a form that is more easily absorbed than iron from foods such as whole grains, pulses, nuts, green leafy vegetables and dried fruit. Iron from these sources is best absorbed when foods rich in vitamin C are eaten at the same meal. Vegetarians who eat a broadly based and well-balanced diet are not usually iron

KEEPING YOUR BLOOD IN GOOD SHAPE

Each red blood cell survives between 100 and 120 days and about 210,000,000,000 red blood cells have to be manufactured each day. To prevent anaemia, your body needs iron, copper, manganese, zinc and vitamins B6, B12, which contains cobalt, and folic acid.

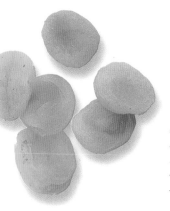

WHEN EXTRA MAY BE NEEDED

• During pregnancy and when breast feeding

• If you regularly take antacid medication for indigestion or stomach ulcers

• By women who have heavy periods, and/or pregnancies close together

• If you drink tea or coffee at mealtimes

• If you are an older person

• If you have previously needed stomach surgery

• If you are on a calorie-restricted diet, especially if you are also a vegetarian

(Pregnant and breast-feeding women should consult a doctor, midwife, or qualified nutritionist before taking any mineral or vitamin supplement.)

LEFT *Dried apricots are a quick and healthy snack and are also a rich source of iron.*

CAN TOO MUCH BE TOXIC?

Too much iron is poisonous, but toxicity is unlikely to be caused by iron from the diet. Iron is stored in the body, and once absorbed it is lost only slowly, except by women of child- bearing years. Fortunately, less than 30 per cent of the iron in food is absorbed, except where

MINERALS

VEGETARIANISM AND IRON
LISA FLETCHER

When Lisa married a vegetarian, she decided that she too would stop eating meat and fish. She was not used to preparing meals without meat and resorted to ready prepared meals, such as vegetable burgers, or cheese dishes, not realizing that the iron she used to consume in red meat wasn't being replaced by these meals. She wasn't getting sufficient iron to replace that lost in the blood during menstruation, and she became very anaemic during her first pregnancy.

The iron tablets that her doctor prescribed caused constipation and abdominal pain, so she did not take the full dose. But after the birth, she felt so exhausted and unwell that her mother-in-law, who was a life-long vegetarian, came to help look after the family. She insisted that Lisa should drink a pint of vegetable juice, sweetened with molasses, each day, and banned tea and coffee altogether for a few weeks. Fruit was eaten at every meal, and Lisa was introduced to a wide variety of dishes containing nuts, seeds and whole grains, as well as cheese and eggs. She began to feel better within a few days and soon learnt how to provide a balanced vegetarian diet.

the anaemia is caused by iron deficiency, when absorption is increased.

However, unnecessary iron supplements taken over a long time can cause damage to the liver and heart, bronzing of the skin and diabetes. There is also some concern that supplements may contribute to atherosclerosis (hardening of the arteries) and heart disease. In addition, iron supplements may reduce the absorption of zinc.

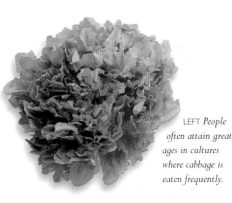

LEFT *People often attain great ages in cultures where cabbage is eaten frequently.*

A GOOD COMBINATION

Adequate supplies of copper, cobalt and manganese in the diet help to ensure that sufficient iron is absorbed.

USING A SUPPLEMENT

Ideally, iron supplements should not be taken at the same time as calcium or zinc supplements, or vitamin E, if the iron is taken as ferrous sulphate (see p49). Iron is best taken between meals with a small dose of vitamin C. If you routinely take a multi-mineral supplement, you should ensure that the iron and zinc that it contains are present in roughly equal amounts.

MINERALS

SUPER NUTRITIOUS OPEN SANDWICHES

• Instead of butter or margarine, spread tahini or hummus on a slice of wholemeal, rye or pumpernickel bread. Then add salad vegetables of your choice and top up with a source of protein such as slices of cold meat, cheese, a hard-boiled egg, one or two sardines, a handful of prawns or chopped nuts, and add the dressing of your choice.

(Note. An increasing number of children are developing sesame seed allergy and, if your family is prone to allergies, mothers may wish to avoid eating sesame seeds in pregnancy or while breast feeding, or giving them to children under three.)

GOOD FOOD SOURCES OF IRON

mg per 100g (3½oz)	
Brewer's yeast	17
Blackstrap molasses	16
Lamb's liver	12
Pumpkin seeds	11
Sesame seeds	11
Tofu	11
Beef liver	9
Soya flour	8
Broad beans	7
Sunflower seeds	7
Dried peaches	7
Dried figs	4
Dried apricots	4
Oatmeal	4
Brazil nuts	3

Cobalt

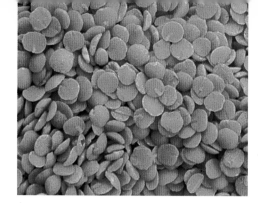

Cobalt is present in the vitamin B12 molecule, and is essential for the manufacture of red blood cells, necessary to prevent anaemia. It does not appear to have any other function.

AVAILABILITY IN FOODS

Provided the diet contains adequate vitamin B12, it is likely to provide enough cobalt (see p27–28). Cobalt is also present in pulses and other vegetables, and may be used by the bacteria in the intestine to make vitamin B12, if this occurs (see vitamin B12).

WHAT IF YOUR INTAKE IS TOO LOW?

See vitamin B12 p27–28.

WHEN EXTRA MAY BE NEEDED

See vitamin B12 p27–28.

CAN TOO MUCH BE TOXIC?

When cobalt was used in the production of beer it was found to damage heart muscle. Cobalt can occur as a food contaminant, and if too much is eaten, it may cause the over-production of red blood cells or damage to the thyroid gland.

A GOOD COMBINATION

See vitamin B12 p27–28.

USING A SUPPLEMENT

This is not recommended.

COBALT, VITAMIN B12 AND ANAEMIA
ANNE GREENE

Anne Greene thought that at 70 she was too young to go into a home. She felt able to look after herself, provided she didn't try to do things in a hurry. It was true that she was a bit short of breath at times, and perhaps a bit unsteady on her feet, which felt as if they were wrapped in cotton wool, but after all, she was getting older.

One evening, she met a neighbour who walked her home. She was very unsteady, and confessed that she found walking much more difficult in the dark than in the light. The neighbour insisted on taking her to the doctor who diagnosed her with pernicious anaemia (see p27–28). She was treated with injections of vitamin B12 and felt very much stronger after a just few weeks.

Zinc

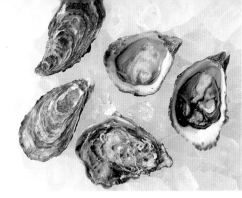

LEFT *Oysters are rich in the zinc needed by men for fertility and normal sexual activity.*

Zinc is essential for a healthy immune system, helping to fight major infections as well as less serious ones, such as boils, acne and sore throats. Without zinc, the body is unable to repair damaged tissues or heal wounds. It plays a major role in cell division, so the tissues that grow throughout life, such as hair, skin and nails, need it to remain healthy. Zinc is also vital for normal growth in children and for their sexual development.

RIGHT *Zinc is one of the many minerals stored in sesame seeds.*

AVAILABILITY IN FOODS

Zinc is present in a wide variety of foods and, like iron, appears to be better absorbed when it comes from animal sources such as muscle meats, fish and seafood. Good vegetable sources include whole grains, nuts, seeds, ginger root and brewer's yeast. Despite being present in so many foods, zinc is often deficient in today's diet because up to 80 per cent of zinc can be lost in the milling process, and it leaches into cooking water. Many soils have become depleted in zinc following the widespread use of chemical fertilizers.

RIGHT *Men need more zinc than women and if they do not obtain enough in their diet, they can be more prone to infection.*

WHAT IF YOUR INTAKE IS TOO LOW?

Serious deficiency leads to a poorly functioning immune system with increased likelihood of infections and allergic conditions, slow healing of wounds, night blindness, loss of smell and taste, falling hair, rashes and other skin problems, white spots on the fingernails, mental lethargy and sleep disturbance. Men may become infertile (see Zinc for men, p76), and periods may be irregular in women. In children, growth may be stunted and sexual maturity delayed.

WHEN EXTRA MAY BE NEEDED

- If you are a man (see Zinc for men p76)
- If you are on a calorie-restricted diet, including slimming or if you are an older person with a small appetite

MINERALS

ZINC FOR MEN

The prostate gland is one of the most zinc-rich organs in the body. The zinc it contains has a role in the control of testosterone production. Zinc deficiency is known to reduce the sperm count, and it is said to be one of the many causes of impotence. It can also cause mental lethargy and emotional problems, leading to a loss of libido.

In older men, there is some evidence that adequate zinc intake may help to avoid problems with the prostate gland, including inflammation and infection. These conditions are difficult to treat with orthodox medicine.

Maintenance of good levels of zinc can be more of a problem for men than women because zinc is needed for the sperm to swim towards the egg for fertilization and so is lost on ejaculation. For this reason, the recommended intake level is higher than for women.

LEFT *Oysters are a very rich source of zinc and would make a healthy treat for a special occasion.*

- At times of particular stress
- If you perspire excessively, and especially if you exercise or take part in sport regularly
- When taking the birth-control pill, diuretics (water tablets) or if you are receiving hormone replacement therapy
- If you regularly drink moderate to large amounts of alcohol, tea or coffee, or smoke
- If you are a vegan or strict vegetarian
- During pregnancy and when breast feeding
- If you have psoriasis (rapid turnover of skin can deplete zinc)

(Pregnant and breast-feeding women should consult a doctor, midwife, or qualified nutritionist before taking any mineral or vitamin supplement.)

CAN TOO MUCH BE TOXIC?

Zinc is relatively non-toxic in doses up to about 100mg, although it may cause some nausea or diarrhoea. Excessive supplementation can cause dizziness, drowsiness and hallucinations.

A GOOD COMBINATION

To be most effective, zinc needs to be accompanied by adequate levels of calcium, copper, phosphorus, selenium and vitamins A, B6 and E

USING A SUPPLEMENT

If you wish to take a supplement, take it at bedtime on an empty stomach, because zinc supplements can interfere with the absorption of other essential minerals, especially iron and copper. If you take a multi-mineral preparation

BELOW *Shrimps and other sea food can contribute to your intake of zinc.*

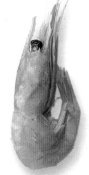

you should ensure that the zinc and iron contained in the supplement are roughly equal in amount.

DID YOU KNOW?

Zinc may be more effective than vitamin C to shorten a cold. Don't swallow zinc tablets whole, but suck them several times a day during the first three or four days of a cold, and not any longer. Some people may experience nausea if they suck these tablets on an empty stomach.

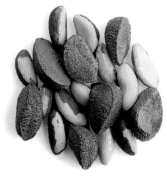

LEFT *Nuts are some of nature's richest foods and Brazil nuts are rich in zinc.*

GOOD FOOD SOURCES OF ZINC	
mg per 100g (3½oz)	
Oysters	50
Sesame seeds	10
Liver	8
Brewer's yeast	8
Pumpkin seeds	7
Shrimps	5
Crab	5
Brazil nuts	5
Beef	4
Cheese	4
Flour (wholemeal)	3
Eggs	1.5
Flour (white)	1

(These figures can vary widely depending on where the plant or animal lived)

MINERALS

MINERALS AND ENERGY
DEBBIE GRANT

Fourteen year-old Debbie Grant was really worried about her schoolwork. She had always been among the top two or three in her class but found that she was becoming too depressed to work as hard as usual, and did not even want to eat. She felt that the only good thing about life was her weight loss, at last she had lost all her 'puppy fat', but she also noted that her periods had stopped.

She had always been what her mother termed a 'picky eater', preferring white bread to brown, and potato crisps to green vegetables. She had become quite a strict vegetarian at 12 and, to keep her mother quiet, she had agreed to take a multi-vitamin supplement. Her mother was afraid that she might be developing anorexia and consulted a friend of the family, who was a nutritionist. They soon realized that Debbie was not eating enough minerals and, in particular, very little zinc at a time when she was growing rapidly.

After taking mineral supplements for a few months, Debbie was back at the top of her class, with plenty of energy. She had even accepted that what she ate could affect her health, and was working hard to eat a balanced diet instead of relying on supplements.

Selenium

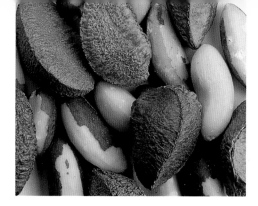

LEFT *Brazil nuts are a rich source of valuable minerals including selenium.*

Selenium has been promoted from being a mineral once regarded as toxic, to one that is listed as essential, albeit in minute quantities. Now hailed as a major anti-ageing mineral, it works with vitamin E to neutralize the dangerous substances known as free radicals, and to eliminate toxic substances, such as cadmium, lead and mercury. Selenium also protects from infection, promotes energy, alleviates menopausal symptoms in women and aids the production of healthy sperm in men. It helps to protect against certain chronic diseases, such as arthritis and multiple sclerosis.

RIGHT *The anti-ageing properties of selenium in combination with vitamin E are now being recognized.*

AVAILABILITY IN FOODS

The selenium that occurs naturally in the soil varies greatly in different parts of the world. Where its occurrence is low, selenium is sometimes included in animal feed. As a result, the amount in our food can vary. Brazil nuts are a particularly rich source, and selenium is found in whole grains and shellfish. Levels of selenium in plants are generally low.

WHAT IF YOUR INTAKE IS TOO LOW?

Selenium deficiency can cause fatigue, increased susceptibility to infection, premature ageing, and loss of fertility, especially in men, and may increase a risk of cancer.

WHEN EXTRA MAY BE NEEDED

- If you live in an area where the soil is deficient in selenium
- If you are a man: like zinc, selenium is lost in seminal fluid
  (Pregnant and breast-feeding women should consult a doctor, midwife, or qualified nutritionist before taking any mineral or vitamin supplement.)

CAN TOO MUCH BE TOXIC?

Selenium is very toxic. Too much selenium can cause hair loss, tooth decay and changes in the nails, including brittleness, pallor, white spots, and even nail loss. The appetite may be poor, with a sour taste in the mouth, and the digestion can become disturbed. Numbness and loss of sensation can occur in the hands and feet. The skin may develop a reddish pigmentation, the breath may smell of a garlic-like odour.

Shampoos containing selenium are used for dandruff and it can be absorbed through the skin in minute quantities. However, it is used here in the form of selenium sulphide, which is less toxic than sodium selenite (see below). Selenium is also used in a number of industrial processes, and can be absorbed by workers in these industries.

RIGHT *Vegetable and animal foods that come from the sea usually contain a rich mix of minerals.*

A GOOD COMBINATION

If you wish to take a selenium supplement, it should always be accompanied by vitamin E.

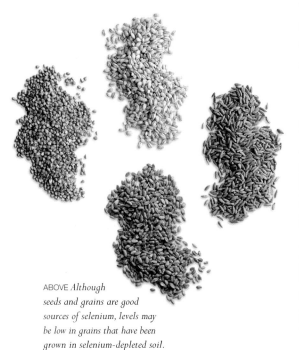

ABOVE *Although seeds and grains are good sources of selenium, levels may be low in grains that have been grown in selenium-depleted soil.*

USING A SUPPLEMENT

Selenium is probably best taken as part of a well-balanced mineral and vitamin programme. The toxicity of selenium appears to vary, depending on the form in which it is taken. Organic selenium (selenocysteine or selenomethionine) is preferable. It is less toxic than sodium selenite, which should not be taken at the same time as vitamin C. If you are sensitive to yeast, it is advisable to check that the brand you are taking is certified as yeast-free, as some selenium supplements may be derived from yeast.

MINERALS

GOOD FOOD SOURCES OF SELENIUM

mcg per 100g (3½oz)

Brazil nuts	102
Scallops	82
Oysters	53
Light molasses	25
Whole grains	12
Eggs	6–60 depending on diet of the hen
Milk	0.5–5 depending on diet of the cow

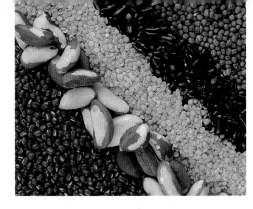

LEFT *Nuts and pulses are actually large seeds, and they are full of minerals in order to provide their new plants with all they need for early growth.*

Copper

Copper is needed in the body, but there is controversy about how much we are receiving. The levels of copper in the soil have been falling, thus reducing the amount available for plants, and many people do not to eat enough of the foods that do contain it. However, the recent widespread use of copper water pipes has raised the possibility that we could be getting too much, especially in a diet that is deficient in zinc. As these two minerals compete for the same pathway into the body, a lack of zinc allows more copper to be absorbed.

deficient anaemia (see p.71). Insufficient copper can increase the likelihood of heart disease, infections, thinning of the bones, and may interfere with the way the nervous system and thyroid gland function.

WHEN EXTRA MAY BE NEEDED

• If you take zinc supplements

(Pregnant and breast-feeding women should consult a doctor, midwife or qualified nutritionist before taking any mineral or vitamin supplement.)

CAN TOO MUCH BE TOXIC?

The symptoms of mild copper toxicity are fatigue, irritability, depression and learning

AVAILABILITY IN FOODS

Copper is present in a wide range of foods including whole grains, seafood, liver, pulses and nuts. It can also come from cooking utensils and water pipes. The absorption of copper into the body can be reduced by the presence of vitamin C, zinc, calcium, manganese, molybdenum, and various toxic substances such as mercury and lead. Copper can be stored in the body, so it is not needed on a daily basis.

WHAT IF YOUR INTAKE IS TOO LOW?

Copper deficiency often occurs alongside iron deficiency, and can increase the severity of iron-

GOOD FOOD SOURCES OF COPPER

mg per 100g (3½oz)	
Oysters	7.6
Lamb's liver	5.5
Brewer's yeast	3.3
Olives	1.6
Dried lentils	0.76
Wholemeal flour	0.4
Walnuts	0.3
Peanuts	0.27
Avocados	0.21
Raw prunes	0.2
Spring onions (scallions)	0.13

RIGHT *White fish, oysters, crabs, lobsters and shrimps all contain useful amounts of copper.*

COPPER BRACELETS: DO THEY WORK?

Although many people claim relief from arthritic pain when they wear a copper bracelet, there is little scientific evidence to support this. It is known that about 13mg of copper is lost each month from one of these bracelets. As not all of this will be absorbed through the skin, bracelets are, at least, unlikely to be harmful. Indeed, one day their mode of action may be discovered. Researchers have shown that a particular form of aspirin, copper salicylate, can provide better pain relief than either copper or aspirin alone.

problems. Excessive intake causes diarrhoea, vomiting, liver damage and discoloration of the skin and hair.

A GOOD COMBINATION

The body makes the best use of copper when there is an adequate supply of cobalt, iron and zinc in the diet.

USING A SUPPLEMENT

Copper supplements on their own are not usually recommended, because toxicity can occur at a relatively low dose. If you wish to take a multi-mineral supplement, it is best to choose one that includes a small amount of copper, to balance the zinc that it contains.

GUACAMOLE

Enjoy the healthy fats found in avocados, and top up your copper at the same time.

SERVES FOUR
2 ripe avocados
juice of 1 lemon or lime
1–2 cloves of garlic, crushed
1–2 spring onions (scallions) sliced finely,
or a small grated onion or shallot
1 large tomato, skinned, seeded and chopped coarsely
½ teaspoon of chilli powder
tabasco sauce to taste
3 tablespoons of chopped coriander (cilantro) leaves
salt and freshly ground pepper to taste

FOR SERVING: Chopped olives and walnuts to garnish, and a selection of raw seasonal vegetables cut into sticks or slices.

METHOD
Peel the avocados and remove the stones. Place the flesh in a large bowl. Add the juice of the lime or lemon. Mash with a fork. Add the other ingredients and taste to check the seasoning.

Serve garnished with the walnuts and olives. Dip the fresh vegetable sticks and slices into the guacamole and enjoy the goodness.

Do not make guacamole too long before you want to serve it, as the avocado may discolour, though this will not affect the flavour.

MINERALS

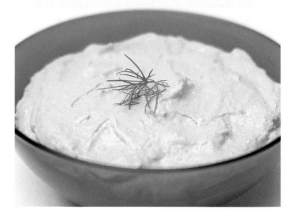

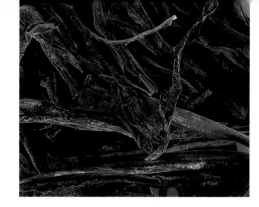

LEFT *Seaweed is a rich, natural source of iodine.*

Iodine

MINERALS

Iodine is a gas, but it is an essential nutrient when dissolved in water. Without iodine the thyroid gland in the neck cannot produce enough of the hormones needed throughout the body, where they help to produce energy from fat, control cholesterol levels and stabilize weight. These hormones aid reproduction, help in the formation of nerves and bone, and keep the skin, nails, hair and teeth in good condition. Iodine also appears to provide some protection against cancers of the breast and uterus (womb).

LEFT *Many aspects of health depend on the thyroid gland being supplied with sufficient iodine.*

AVAILABILITY IN FOODS

The amount of iodine in the average diet varies widely from area to area. It depends on the amount of iodine in the soil, the diet of animals farmed for milk, eggs or meat, and the amount of sea fish, sea vegetables, such as kelp (see p96), and sea salt that are eaten. Iodine is also used industrially in colouring dyes and dough conditioners, so it is possible that you are eating more than you realize. As iodine is not stored in the body, a regular intake is essential.

WHAT IF YOUR INTAKE IS TOO LOW?

When iodine is deficient in the diet, the thyroid gland enlarges to maximize its uptake of iodine from the blood. This is known as goitre. Even this enlargement may not allow the gland to produce sufficient thyroid hormones, and long-term deficiency can cause obesity, constipation, weakness, mental slowness and, eventually, insanity.

WHEN EXTRA MAY BE NEEDED

- If the iodine level in the soil is low, and you do not eat sea fish or sea vegetables
- During pregnancy and when breast feeding
- If you eat a salt-reduced diet
  (Pregnant and breast-feeding women should consult a doctor, midwife, or qualified nutritionist before taking any mineral or vitamin supplement.)

CAN TOO MUCH BE TOXIC?

Toxicity is unlikely from iodine obtained from natural dietary sources eaten in normal quantities, as it is rapidly eliminated from the body. However, supplementation with too much commercially iodized salt or kelp products may produce skin rashes and aggravate acne. Very high levels can, paradoxically, cause goitre and reduce the output of the thyroid gland. These effects were found in a group of Japanese fishermen who were absorbing up to 30,000–100,000mcg of iodine each day from eating seaweed. Skin contact with iodine can cause dermatitis in some people.

A GOOD COMBINATION

No information is available.

USING A SUPPLEMENT

Ideally, we should obtain adequate iodine from food and, where desired, sea salt seasoning. This contains less iodine than commercially iodized salt, which is not recommended, as it contains aluminium and other chemicals. Moderate amounts of kelp powder (see p96) or tablets can also be used. Multi-mineral tablets usually contain iodine at a moderate level.

GOOD FOOD SOURCES OF IODINE

mcg per 100g (3½oz)	
Haddock	200
Cod	100
Cheese	50
Herring	25
Fruits, vegetables, cereals and meats	10

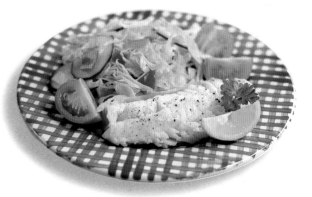

ABOVE *Sea fish, such as haddock, can be a major source of iodine in your diet.*

MINERALS

SEAWEED AS FOOD

Although seaweed has been eaten for thousands of years, it is likely that its usefulness is only just being fully explored. Seaweed has a variety of industrial uses, and has long been used in more than one type of traditional or folk medicine to cure a wide variety of illnesses. All types of seaweed contain plentiful iodine, some are able to inhibit viruses, including the herpes and AIDS viruses, while others show anti-cancer potential.

The brown types of dried seaweed that are now widely available in health food stores and oriental food outlets include wakame, which is used in miso soup, kombu and arame. Red seaweed used as food include nori, often used to wrap sushi, agar-agar, dulse and Irish moss.

RIGHT *Kelp supplements are made from brown seaweed.*

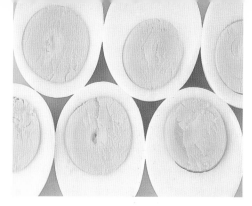

LEFT *Egg yolks are a rich source of chromium and can usually be easily introduced into most people's diets.*

Chromium

Chromium is needed by the body in extremely small quantities. Even these small quantities are often not available from the refined diet that is common in developed countries. For example, it has been estimated that up to 50 per cent of Americans eat a diet that is deficient in chromium. By stabilizing the level of glucose in the blood, chromium helps to regulate the levels of cholesterol and other fats. It appears to act by stimulating the pancreas to produce more insulin, and by improving the action of insulin in the blood.

MINERALS

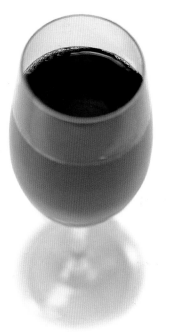

AVAILABILITY IN FOODS

Chromium is present in beef, egg yolks, whole grains and many vegetables, including potato skins. Brewer's yeast and molasses (see p26) are also excellent sources of chromium, but torula yeast contains very little. Up to half the daily requirement for chromium may be obtained from the water in hard water areas. Chromium is poorly absorbed into the body, especially in elderly people and when milk or other foods that are high in phosphorus (see p58 and p63) or fat are eaten at the same time.

WHAT IF YOUR INTAKE IS TOO LOW?

Insufficient chromium in the diet is thought to be partly responsible for the development of late-onset diabetes, for raised cholesterol levels, obesity and atherosclerosis (hardening of the arteries). Even mild deficiency may cause abnormalities in blood sugar levels that can result in anxiety or fatigue. Deficiencies are most common in older people and in the young, especially teenagers on poor diets.

WHEN EXTRA MAY BE NEEDED

• If you are overweight
• If your cholesterol level is high
• If you exercise or train regularly, as chromium is then lost in the urine

LEFT *A glass of either red or white wine is a congenial source of chromium.*

LEFT *Choose wholemeal bread in preference to white bread, which contains very little chromium.*

- If your diet contains a high proportion of refined food like white bread and flour, fat and sugar
- If you are prone to low blood-sugar levels, including the sugar craving that can occur in pre-menstrual syndrome
- During pregnancy

  (*Pregnant and breast-feeding women should consult a doctor, midwife, or qualified nutritionist before taking any mineral or vitamin supplement.*)

CAN TOO MUCH BE TOXIC?

Since chromium is poorly absorbed and excreted easily, toxicity is unlikely, even when it is taken as a supplement.

A GOOD COMBINATION

The absorption of chromium is thought to be enhanced by the presence of vitamin B3, and the amino acids glycine, cysteine, and glutamic acid (see Glucose Tolerance Factor).

USING A SUPPLEMENT

Chromium appears to be best absorbed when taken as glucose tolerance factor(see Glucose Tolerance Factor), or as chromium picolinate. Supplements that are derived from yeast sources should be avoided if you are sensitive to yeast.

GLUCOSE TOLERANCE FACTOR

Chromium is an essential part of the molecule that has been called 'glucose tolerance factor' (GTF) or polynicotinate. The exact chemical structure of GTF is unknown but, in addition to chromium, it contains vitamin B3 and the amino acids glycine, cysteine, and glutamic acid.

GTF occurs naturally in brewer's yeast, and is now available as a dietary supplement. It has been used successfully to ease the sugar cravings of pre-menstrual syndrome.

So far, there is little evidence that GTF can help people with established diabetes, but research is continuing. If you have diabetes you should consult your doctor before taking GTF, in case your dose of medication has to be changed.

Elderly people, who have marginally raised blood glucose levels and are at risk of developing diabetes do appear to benefit from GTF. It has been shown that supplements can improve the way that glucose levels are controlled.

MINERALS

GOOD FOOD SOURCES OF CHROMIUM

mcg per 100g (3½oz)	
Egg yolk	183
Molasses	121
Brewer's yeast	117
Beef	57
Wine	45
Wholemeal bread	42
Rye bread	30
Old potatoes	27

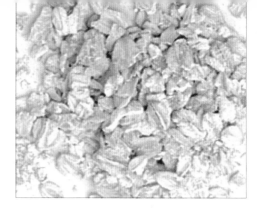

LEFT *Whole grains, such as oatflakes, are good sources of manganese.*

Manganese

Manganese is an underrated, but essential, trace mineral. It enables the body to make effective use of vitamins C, B1, biotin and choline. Without manganese the body cannot make fat, sex hormones or, in women, breast milk. It appears to help the body to neutralize the damaging substances known as free radicals, to prevent diabetes and to preserve normal nerve function.

MINERALS

AVAILABILITY IN FOODS

As with iron, absorption of manganese is poor, with only about 15–30 per cent of intake being used by the body. However, it is widely available in plant foods, including nuts, whole grains, pulses, leafy greens, especially spinach and alfalfa (see p98), tea and coffee. Up to 90 per cent of manganese in whole grains is lost during milling. Its absorption into the body can be reduced by the simultaneous intake of large amounts of calcium (high in milk), phosphorus (high in meats and fizzy drinks), zinc, cobalt and soy protein. It competes for the same absorption pathway as iron: either mineral when taken in large amounts will inhibit the absorption of the other. The level of manganese in the soil can be depleted by the use of chemical fertilizers, or made unavailable to plants by over-use of lime.

WHAT IF YOUR INTAKE IS TOO LOW?

Manganese deficiency is rare. Symptoms include poor growth of bones, problems with cartilage and the discs between the vertebrae (bones in the spine), alterations in brain and muscle function, birth defects, reduced control of glucose levels in the blood, hearing problems and reduced fertility. Serious deficiencies in infants can cause paralysis, convulsions, blindness and deafness.

WHEN EXTRA MAY BE NEEDED

• While breast feeding
• If you take calcium or phosphorus supplements *(Pregnant and breast-feeding women should consult a doctor, midwife, or qualified nutritionist before taking any mineral or vitamin supplement.)*

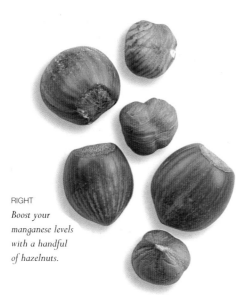

RIGHT
Boost your manganese levels with a handful of hazelnuts.

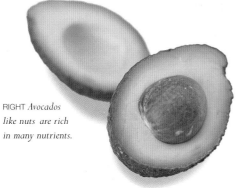

RIGHT *Avocados like nuts are rich in many nutrients.*

CAN TOO MUCH BE TOXIC?

Although manganese appears to be relatively non-toxic when eaten, a condition that is sometimes known as 'manganese madness' occurs in those who work in manganese mines and inhale it.

A GOOD COMBINATION

The body uses manganese most effectively in the presence of vitamins B1 and E, and calcium and phosphorus.

USING A SUPPLEMENT

Manganese is best taken as part of a well-balanced mineral and vitamin supplement.

GOOD FOOD SOURCES OF MANGANESE

	mg per 100g (3½oz)
Wheat flour	6
Oatflakes	4.9
Wholemeal bread	4.3
Avocados	4.2
Hazelnuts	3.5
Buckwheat flour	2.1
Peas	2
Olives	1.2

TABBOULEH

There are many variations to this dish which originated in the Middle East. You can vary the ingredients according to season and your personal taste, and use it as the main dish or as a side dish.

200g (7oz) bulgar wheat (or left-over pre-cooked whole grains such as rice, quinoa, or millet)
100g (3½oz) parsley or more if you wish
10 spring onions (scallions)
1 or more cloves of garlic, finely chopped
1 tablespoon chopped mint or coriander (cilantro)
1 large tomato, seeded and chopped

DRESSING
3 tablespoonfuls of lemon, lime or grapefruit juice
2 tablespoonfuls of olive oil, or other oil of your choice

METHOD
Cover the bulgar wheat with boiling water and allow it to stand for 30 minutes while you prepare the other ingredients. Then squeeze out any excess water and place the bulgar wheat in the salad bowl. If using the other grains, simply place them in the bowl.

Add the other ingredients to the wheat and mix together thoroughly.

Combine the dressing ingredients, add to the tabbouleh and toss.

Serve chilled.

(Variants: you can add chopped chicken or turkey, crumbled feta or other cheese, chopped nuts or hard-boiled eggs, other vegetables such as grated carrots, chopped peppers, or cooked beans or chickpeas (garbanzo beans).

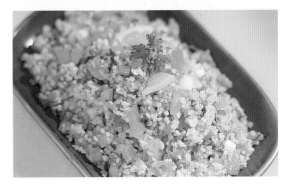

Molybdenum

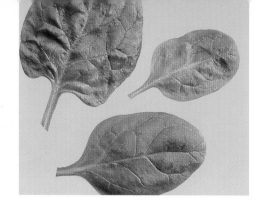

LEFT *Spinach and other dark green leafy vegetables will help you to increase your intake of molybdenum.*

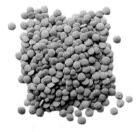

Although molybdenum is only required in minute amounts, it can be low in the diet as a result of poor levels in the soil and food processing. It protects the body from nitrosamines, chemicals that are associated with cancer of the oesophagus (gullet), and which are found in the soil when molybdenum is at a low level. Nitrosamines have also been found in the bowel after foods containing nitrites and nitrates (used as preservatives in hot dogs, luncheon meat and similar meat products), have been eaten. Molybdenum may also help to prevent anaemia.

AVAILABILITY IN FOODS

Molybdenum is found in whole grains, brewer's yeast, pulses, dark green leafy vegetables and in liver and other organ meats, but it is lost in the milling process. It competes with copper for absorption into the body.

RIGHT *Lentils are a cook's dream food: rich in nutrients — they don't require soaking and are cooked within 20 minutes.*

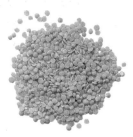

WHAT IF YOUR INTAKE IS TOO LOW?

Information about deficiency is limited, although it may lead to visual problems, palpitations and diminished consciousness. In a few people, low molybdenum intake can cause sensitivity to sulphite preservatives, resulting in nausea, diarrhoea and asthma.

WHEN EXTRA MAY BE NEEDED

- If you eat a refined, junk-food diet
- If you take copper supplements *(Pregnant and breast-feeding women should consult a doctor, midwife, or qualified nutritionist before taking any mineral or vitamin supplement.)*

MOLYDBENUM AND CANCER

In the Lin Xian region of China, poor levels of molybdenum in the soil, combined with a low vitamin C intake, resulted in the highest rate of oesophageal (gullet) cancer in the world. Although there is no evidence that supplementary molybdenum will protect against cancer, it is possible that enrichment of the soil, where it is deficient, might do so.

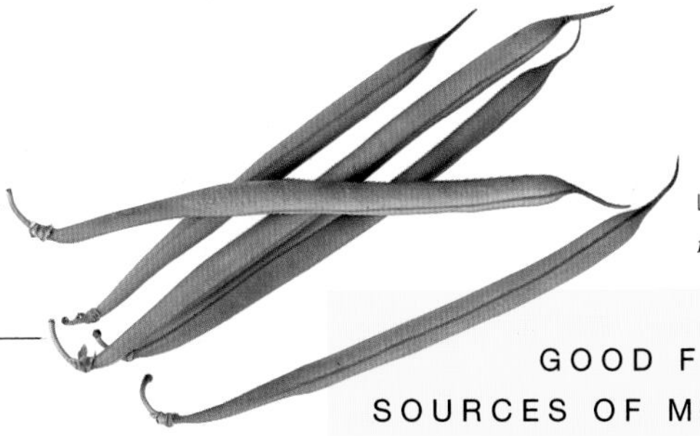

LEFT *Green beans contain a rich array of nutrients.*

CAN TOO MUCH BE TOXIC?

It is possible that high molybdenum intake may cause gouty arthritis. In animals, high levels seems to cause loss of appetite, and a shorter life span.

A GOOD COMBINATION

No information is available.

USING A SUPPLEMENT

If you wish to take a supplement, it should be taken as part of a well-balanced multi-vitamin and mineral supplement that also contains copper.

GOOD FOOD SOURCES OF MOLYBDENUM

mcg per 100g (3½oz)	
Buckwheat	485
Lima beans	400
Wheat germ	200
Lentils	120
Sunflower seeds	103
Kidney	75
Green beans	66
Eggs	50

MINERALS

GLORIOUS GRAINS

Grains have played an important part in our diet for over 10,000 years. They are rich sources of starch, fibre and, apart from the outer bran coverings, usually contain an excellent supply of minerals and vitamins. However, we do seem to be very dependent on wheat and many people are becoming intolerant of wheat. It is a good idea to eat a wide variety of different grains when possible, including:

Amaranth contains plenty of protein, including lysine, an essential amino acid that is often absent from other grains, most of the B-vitamins, fibre, calcium and iron. Whole grains can be toasted before being cooked like rice.

Barley is mostly used in soups, but barley bread was once very popular. When whole, it contains 10–15 per cent of protein, B-vitamins, especially B3 and folic acid, and magnesium, calcium, iron, phosphorus and potassium.

Buckwheat is not wheat at all, and can be eaten by those who are intolerant of wheat. It is generally grown without fertilizers and contains all the amino acids that we need, plus B-vitamins, plenty of potassium, and some iron, calcium, manganese and phosphorus. The grain can be cooked as porridge and it is also available as flour or pasta.

Millet is a gluten-free grain. Both tasty and nourishing, it contains 15 per cent of protein, vitamins B1, B2, and B3, some vitamin E, and is rich in iron, potassium and calcium. The whole grain can be toasted, then cooked in water and used in the same way as rice.

Quinoa can be substituted for meat as it contains all the amino acids that we need and is rich in iron. It also contains a range of B-vitamins, and calcium. Like rice, it should be rinsed before being cooked in water, which takes 15–20 minutes.

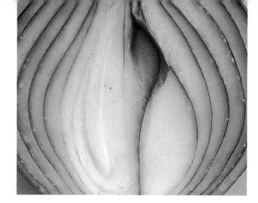

LEFT *In addition to silicon, onions contain many medicinal compounds.*

Silicon

Although silicon is the most abundant mineral in the earth's crust, very little is actually present in the human body. All the same, it is found in virtually every tissue, especially the hair (where it may inhibit greying), the nails and the skin (where it maintains strength with suppleness). Silicon also keeps the bones, cartilage, tendons and artery walls strong. Currently being further investigated, it is a mineral that is said to be beneficial for many conditions including heartburn and dyspepsia, allergies and gum disease.

AVAILABILITY IN FOODS

Silicon is found in plant fibres especially in whole grains, such as wheat, oats, millet, barley and rice, as well as in onions, beetroot, alfalfa (see p98), and horsetail (see p95). It is also present in hard water.

WHAT IF YOUR INTAKE IS TOO LOW?

There is little information available, but deficiency may affect bone and tooth structure. It may be one factor among many that increases the risk of heart disease and atherosclerosis (hardening of the arteries). There is some evidence that lack of silica in the tissues is associated with poor stamina.

WHEN EXTRA MAY BE NEEDED

At present there is no clear evidence of deficiency.

CAN TOO MUCH BE TOXIC?

No information is currently available.

A GOOD COMBINATION

No information is currently available.

USING A SUPPLEMENT

Various plant derivatives are available for supplemental use, and they can be bought in many forms, such as tablets, capsules, powders and gels. You should follow any instructions on the bottle.

LEFT *Beetroot is an underrated vegetable that contains many useful minerals.*

SILICONE IMPLANTS

Silicon is sometimes confused with silicone. However, silicon (also sometimes called silica) is a naturally occurring substance that differs considerably from silicone, which has been used in breast implants. Silicone is an industrial polymer, which appears to cause severe symptoms in some women, and may be a cause of cancer.

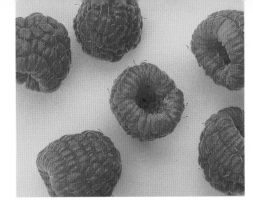

LEFT *Raspberries are a summer treat — low in calories but rich in nutrients.*

Sulphur

Sulphur is a non-metallic element that is often not listed as 'essential' because there are no specific deficiency symptoms. However, our bodies contain as much sulphur as potassium. It has been called the beauty mineral as it is found in skin, hair and nails. It helps to detoxify the body, boost the immune system and counteract the effects of ageing and the diseases of older age, such as arthritis. Sulphur is an essential constituent of protein, biotin and vitamin B1.

AVAILABILITY IN FOODS

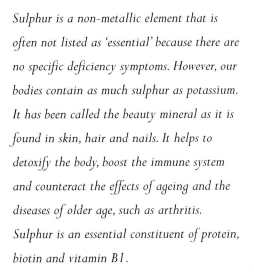

Sulphur is found in protein foods, especially egg yolks, garlic, lettuce, raspberries and the brassica family, such as cabbage, turnip, kale and Brussels sprouts. It is the hydrogen sulphide in onions that makes us weep while chopping them.

ABOVE *Onions are among the many plants that contain plenty of sulphur.*

WHAT IF YOUR INTAKE IS TOO LOW?

Insufficient sulphur is only likely to occur in those who have a very low protein intake (during illness or, possibly, as a result of a poorly planned strict vegan diet). The main concern would then be lack of protein rather than lack of sulphur.

WHEN EXTRA MAY BE NEEDED

Sulphur deficiency does not occur in isolation, but may be associated with protein deficiency.

CAN TOO MUCH BE TOXIC?

Toxicity has not been reported.

A GOOD COMBINATION

Sulphur is best used with the B-vitamins.

USING A SUPPLEMENT

As extra sulphur is readily available in food, a supplement is not necessary.

MINERALS

GOOD FOOD SOURCES OF SULPHUR

	mg per 100g (3½oz)
Shellfish	250–450
Nuts	150–380
Garlic	370
Meats	200–330
Cheese	240
Eggs	180
Indian tea	180
Cooked Brussels sprouts	78
Raw onions	51
Raspberries	17

Herbal helpers

In the 2,000 years since Hippocrates urged that our food should be our medicine and medicine should be our food, the medical profession has tried hard to prove him wrong and has introduced many non-food medicines. Today, however, the pharmaceutical industry is looking increasingly towards plants as sources of new medicines and there is a growing awareness that plants can prevent ill-health and even heal in some cases.

The World Health Organization recommends that we should eat at least five portions of fruit and vegetables each day. Many of these have medicinal effects that are so gentle we are hardly aware of them. Scientific understanding of the way that fruit and vegetables contribute to health is still very sketchy. However, there is a growing awareness that food can indeed be a medicine and research is continuing. Some of the plants known to have particular beneficial effects are described in this section.

Non-culinary herbs have probably always been used as medicines. A few of those that can now be bought as proprietary preparations are also described here. They are available in pharmacies and health food shops, and their effect can be powerful. They should, like all medicines, be used with caution and treated with respect.

The advice given here is not intended to replace professional advice from your doctor or qualified herbalist, but merely to supplement it.

RIGHT *The medicinal qualities of herbs have long been recognized and herbs are now available in easy-to-take forms such as tablets.*

USING HERBS SAFELY

- Never exceed the manufacturer's recommended dose
- Stop taking your herbal medicine if you suffer side-effects
- Always seek professional advice if your symptoms persist
- Do not take herbal medicines in pregnancy or when breast feeding, unless their safety has been established
- If you are taking conventional medicine, or have any long-term medical condition, check with your doctor before taking a herbal medicine or supplement

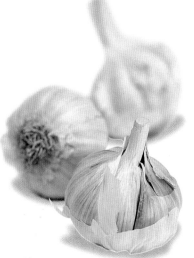

Allium sativum
Garlic

Garlic appears to act as a natural antibiotic and anti-fungal agent, but it may also stimulate the immune system. It has been used externally to alleviate superficial infections. Long-term internal use of garlic may help to prevent heart disease by lowering cholesterol and reducing the stickiness of the blood. It appears to regulate blood-sugar levels and may even prevent tumours.

Fresh garlic is probably the best source of the active ingredients; deodorized commercial preparations may be less effective. Fresh parsley reduces the smell of garlic on the breath. Breast-feeding mothers may find that their babies dislike the taste of garlic in breast milk.

CAUTION

• Large amounts of garlic can cause heartburn, especially during pregnancy
• Fresh garlic can cause local irritation and ulceration if left in contact with skin or mucous membranes

Aloe vera
Aloe vera

The popularity of aloe vera has far outstripped the ability of scientists to verify the many health claims that have been made for it. Gel from the leaves has been used for over 2,000 years to reduce the discomfort of burns, ulcers, eczema and other skin conditions, and it may also accelerate healing.

When taken orally, aloe vera is said to soothe inflammation in the digestive system, relieve irritable bowel syndrome (IBS) and other bowel disorders. It appears to have little toxicity, but if you have a serious bowel disorder or an immune deficiency disease such as AIDS, it would be wise to consult your doctor before using it.

Aloe vera is widely available as a gel or ointment, and for oral use.

HERBAL
HELPERS

CAUTION

• High doses of aloe vera can cause vomiting and diarrhoea
• Occasionally, a reaction may develop on hypersensitive skin

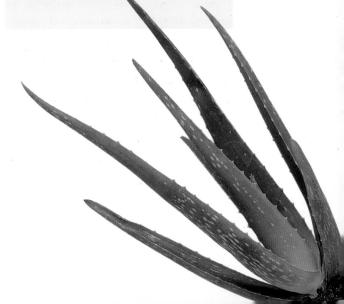

Avena sativa

Oats

Oatmeal porridge has long been known to soothe the digestive system and reduce constipation. You can make a soothing bath for dry or eczematous skin by suspending a small bag of oatmeal under the hot tap when the bath is being filled. Oats also contain substances that protect against certain cancers.

The soluble fibre found in oats slows the digestion of starchy foods and gives the body better control of the level of sugar in the blood. People who need to inject insulin can sometimes reduce the dose by eating more soluble fibre. Steadier blood-sugar levels often reduce hunger and improve weight control.

Recently, it has been shown that oat bran supplements help to lower the level of cholesterol in the blood. They should be introduced gradually to the diet to give the digestive system time to adjust.

CAUTION

• Avoid if you are sensitive to gluten

Capsicum frutescens / annum

Cayenne chilli

Fresh chilli peppers are packed with beta-carotene and vitamin C, and can act in many other ways to combat ill health. Chilli peppers may protect against heart attacks and strokes by stimulating the circulation, by making the blood less likely to clot, and by reducing cholesterol levels in the blood. They relieve congestion from colds and may improve digestion. The heat produced by chilli peppers induces sweating and speeds up the chemical processes of the body. This combats chills and may aid weight loss.

Chilli peppers have been used for many centuries to relieve pain. When eaten, they release endorphins, the natural pain-relieving substances produced in the brain. Excessive heat can be countered with a banana or glass of milk.

CAUTION

• Avoid touching eyes or cuts after handling chilli peppers
• Consult your doctor before taking medicinal doses

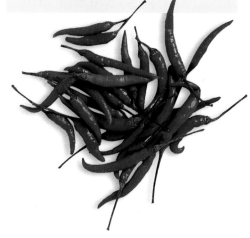

Echinacea spp.
Echinacea

Used in Native American medicine, members of the Echinacea *family have become popular home remedies to combat infection, especially by those who wish to avoid taking antibiotics.*

Echinacea herbs appear to stimulate certain parts of the immune system (the macrophages and natural killer cells) to overcome bacteria, fungi, including vaginal thrush, and viruses, such as herpes. They may even, one day, be found to have a role in combating tumour cells.

The long-term effects on the immune system are not known and it is probably best to avoid taking Echinacea for more than two or three weeks at any one time. If you have any deficiency of your immune system, consult your doctor as there have been reports that other parts of the immune system (the T4 helper cells) have occasionally been suppressed in people taking Echinacea.

CAUTION

- Exceeding the recommended dose may cause nausea and dizziness
- Avoid if you have multiple sclerosis

Equisetum spp.
Horsetail

Horsetail is a rich source of silica and has been taken as a herbal supplement to promote the health of the skin and blood vessels, and to strengthen the bones, teeth and hair. It also provides other minerals, including calcium, copper and zinc.

Horsetail acts as a mild diuretic, and has been used to relieve disorders of the prostate. It was used by the ancient Greeks for the treatment of wounds and in folk medicines as a general tonic. Herbalists still use it to control bleeding. It is said to remove white spots from fingernails, probably because it contains a good supply of zinc (see p75). Horsetail is available in tablets and capsules.

CAUTION

- As with all supplements, do not exceed the recommended dose

HERBAL
HELPERS

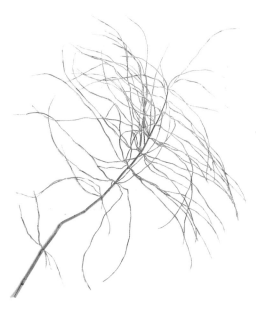

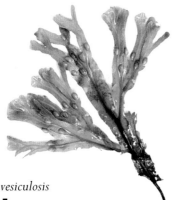

Fucus vesiculosis
Kelp

*Several varieties of seaweed are used in commercial kelp preparations, one of the commonest being bladderwrack (*Fucus vesiculosis*). Kelp has been used for over 200 years in the treatment of goitre, as it is a major source of iodine (see p82). It also contains other minerals, including calcium, magnesium and potassium, and vitamins, such as B3, B2 riboflavin, and choline.*

Kelp is frequently taken as a health-food supplement either in tablet form or as a powder, which can be used (in moderation) as a salt substitute. In addition to providing iodine, kelp may prevent the absorption of toxic metals that can occur in small quantities in the diet. It has mild anti-rheumatic properties, for which it may also be applied externally. If you collect your own kelp for external use, always take it from the sea, rather than the beach. Avoid areas of industrial pollution, as kelp can be contaminated by heavy metals, such as cadmium and mercury.

CAUTION

- As with all supplements, do not exceed the recommended dose

Hydrastis canadensis
Goldenseal

Goldenseal was used by the Native Americans to treat many ailments, especially infections. Modern analysis has shown that it contains substances that fight many types of infection including those caused by bacteria, parasites, yeasts and worms. It appears to stimulate the immune system and may have some anti-tumour properties.

Goldenseal is particularly useful for conditions that affect the mucous membranes, such as colds and other catarrhal conditions. The dose recommended by the manufacturer can be taken for two or three weeks, but longer courses may cause liver irritation. Herbalists sometimes recommend weak solutions of goldenseal as douches for vaginal discharge, but medical diagnosis is essential if the condition persists.

CAUTION

- Avoid if you are pregnant or have raised blood pressure
- The fresh herb can cause mouth ulcers

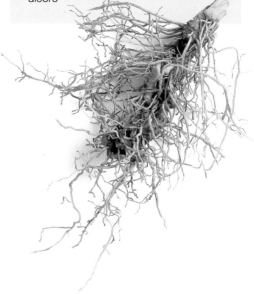

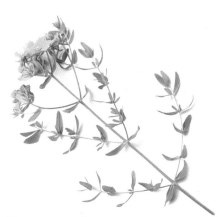

Hypericum perforatum
St John's wort

St John's wort has been used as a medicinal herb since at least the times of the Crusades, when it was used to help heal battle wounds. Modern chemical assessment has confirmed that it has anti-viral and anti-bacterial properties, and it may have a role in the treatment of AIDS. It has been used to relieve coughs and neuralgia, including sciatica. However, its most popular use today is in the treatment of depression and for the relief of long-standing nervous exhaustion. Its effectiveness has been confirmed by many clinical and laboratory studies.

If you are already taking anti-depressant medication, you should consult your doctor before taking St John's wort. It is widely available in tablet or capsule form.

CAUTION

- The skin may become sensitive to sunlight
- Touching the fresh herb can cause skin eruptions

Glycyrrhiza glabra
Liquorice

Liquorice confectionery rarely contains any extract from the herb. Herbal liquorice has wide medicinal action and its sweetness makes it acceptable to children. It appears to act both as a laxative and like a mild cortisone, which is an essential hormone with a wide area of activity in the body.

Liquorice soothes coughs, while promoting the expulsion of phlegm. It aids the healing of stomach and duodenal ulcers, relieves arthritis by its anti-inflammatory action, fights infection and may protect against the formation of tumours. In women, liquorice is said to regulate periods and may even increase fertility. Laboratory tests undertaken so far have shown that it may have powerful anti-viral activity against the AIDS and herpes viruses, but further research is needed.

In healthy people, liquorice appears to be safe when taken for short periods in the doses recommended by the manufacturer. However, it can cause water retention and you should seek medical advice if you have heart disease, including high blood pressure, kidney or liver disease.

CAUTION

- Avoid if you are taking digoxin or related drugs

HERBAL HELPERS

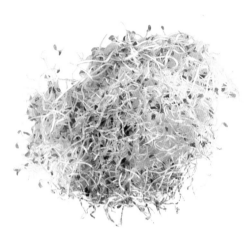

Medicago sativa
Alfalfa

The main benefit of alfalfa is as a food supple-ment. Rich in beta-carotene, vitamins C, D, E and several of the B-vitamins, it is also one of the rare plants that contain vitamin K. Alfalfa roots can penetrate the soil by up to 33m (100ft), enabling the plant to build up a rich store of minerals including iron, phosphorus, magnesium, calcium, potassium and silicon.

Alfalfa is reputed to reduce heart disease and prevent fluid retention. It may help to protect against tumours and viral infection.

Alfalfa is available in tablet form and as sprouts (see p35), and it appears to be a generally very safe supplement.

CAUTION

- Alfalfa can aggravate systemic lupus erythematosis, an inflammatory disease

Tanacetum parthenium
Feverfew

Feverfew has been used for centuries to relieve headaches and migraines. It can be taken regularly as a preventive measure, or when the headache occurs. Several different prepa-rations are available and the strength of these may vary. If you grow feverfew, you may wish to use fresh leaves although they often cause mouth ulcers. These can be avoided if the leaves are eaten as a small sandwich with bread, or fried in a little oil.

Feverfew may also relieve the inflammation of arthritis, and possibly other similar diseases.

Although feverfew appears to be non-toxic, some experts advise taking it regularly for no more than two weeks, and then restarting when symptoms recur.

CAUTION

- Avoid if you take anti-coagulant (blood thinning) medication

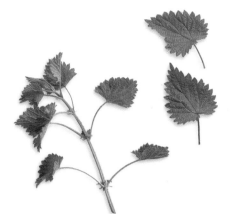

Urtica urens or dioica

The common nettle

The Romans are said to have imported their own nettles to Britain because they thought the glowing sensation from nettle stings on their skin would help them to keep warm. In some parts of the world, nettles are still used in this way to alleviate the pain of rheumatism. More acceptable, perhaps, is the use of nettle infusions by herbal practitioners to treat arthritis. They may also help eczema, and enhance the flow of milk of breast-feeding mothers.

You can treat yourself to a spring tonic by eating very young leaves. They are rich in potassium, iron, calcium, silicon, and vitamins A and C. Cook and use them in the same way as spinach, or wilt them fairly briefly and use in salads. Once cooked, nettles no longer sting.

CAUTION

- Choose a pollution-free area for harvesting young nettle shoots

Zingiber officinale

Ginger

Ginger grows in the wild in Asia and was introduced to northern Europe by the Romans. Medicinal ginger is derived from the root of the plant and has been used as a digestive aid for at least 2,000 years. It stimulates the appetite, relieves nausea and travel sickness, and assists in the expulsion of wind. It has been used to relieve the nausea of pregnancy, and appears to be safe when taken in moderate amounts.

Ginger aids digestion by stimulating the appetite, and relieving nausea and travel sickness. It stimulates the circulation and, in warming the body, promotes sweating. It may reduce the risk of heart disease and make the blood less sticky. A compress made from ginger-root tea can relieve tired and aching muscles by stimulating the blood supply.

HERBAL HELPERS

CAUTION

- Avoid if you have a stomach or duodenal ulcer

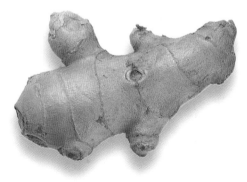

Your special needs

In developed countries today, many people complain of being 'tired all the time' or 'stressed out'. All too often their difficulties are caused by the inferior quality of their diets, for food is the fuel that keeps our 'engines' going. Banish feeling under the weather by treating yourself to a healthy diet, supplemented if necessary by the vitamins, minerals and herbs suggested in this chapter and chosen by you to suit your age and lifestyle. Remember: eating a healthy diet does not mean that you can't indulge yourself occasionally; just don't do it all the time!

YOUR
SPECIAL
NEEDS

Food is, of course, more than just fuel. Eating can also be fun and we celebrate religious, national and personal events with festive meals. There is no real problem if these meals are less than perfect nutritionally, but an inadequate diet on all the other days of the year will, in the long run, lead to poor performances at work and play, indifferent health and even illness.

During the early years of life, the growing body needs a plentiful supply of protein, vitamins and minerals and, for growth to take place, there has to be a relatively high input of calories.

Once growth is complete, fewer calories are needed, but the requirement for vitamins and minerals remains the same as during adolescence. This creates a problem because the lower intake of food makes it difficult to obtain sufficient minerals and vitamins from the diet. This problem is compounded by the lower calorie needs of modern adults whose lives are more sedentary than at any time in the past. Adults, therefore, have little leeway for eating so-called 'empty calories', that is, calories that come from food such as refined flours and sugar, in which other nutrients are at a low level or even absent.

A nutritionally rich diet becomes even more important when the normal events of adult life, such as parenthood, injuries, surgery and stressful jobs, increase the body's need for

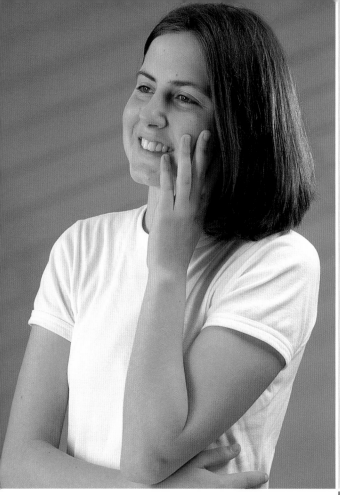

SIX IMPORTANT NUTRIENTS

1. CARBOHYDRATES These provide starches and sugars needed for energy.

2. PROTEINS These build body tissues during growth and repair them later in life.

3. FATS These are needed to maintain cell walls throughout the body, including the brain and skin.

4. MINERALS These are needed for structure and to maintain fluid distribution in the body.

5. VITAMINS These are needed to control the basic functions of the body.

6. WATER Essential for the maintenance of life.

vitamins and minerals. In addition, good nutrition can help to prevent heart disease and may reduce the risk of developing cancer.

In later years, nutritional needs change again in small but significant ways. Older people gradually become less active, reducing calorie requirements even further, yet vitamin and mineral needs remain unchanged. In addition, poor appetite and lack of energy to buy and cook food can reduce the intake of nutrients at a time when the body may be becoming less efficient in the way it uses them.

This chapter offers guidance on how to ensure that nutritional needs for different lifestyles can be met throughout life for the maintenance of good health. Special needs are recognized and further information on the recommended vitamins, minerals and herbs can be found in the first three chapters of this book.

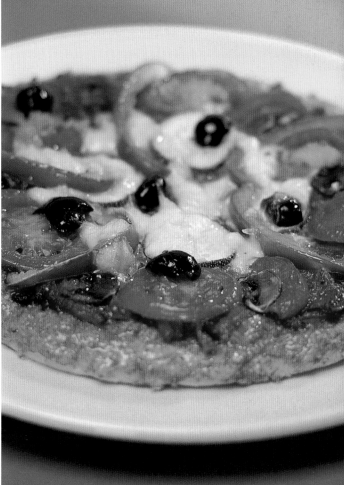

The first two years

A baby clearly needs good nutrition if it is to grow and stay healthy. With the increase in our nutritional knowledge, we are becoming ever more aware that good nutrition plays a major part in the development of the brain, the learning of skills and the effective functioning of the different systems of the body, such as the glands that produce hormones. While we cannot replace the natural goodness of a mother's milk, there is much we can do to replicate it.

YOUR
SPECIAL
NEEDS

Nourishment from milk

In the first few days after her baby's birth, the mother produces breast milk known as colostrum. This milk is rich in zinc and other nutrients needed to enhance the baby's immune system, which is coming into contact with infection for the first time.

After a few days, the fat and vitamin E in the milk are increased to feed the fatty tissues of the brain and strengthen the baby's immune system. Later, the milk will contain more of the protein and carbohydrate needed for growth and energy. The content of breast milk can change during a single feed to ensure that the nutrients most needed are provided in the early stages before the baby tires. A well-nourished mother can usually provide all the nutrients needed by her baby during the first six months of life.

Fortunately, we are now able to analyze breast milk, and this knowledge has been used to improve the quality of infant milk formulas needed by the five per cent of babies whose mothers are unable to breast feed them.

When to wean

The increasing numbers of small children with allergic conditions and digestive difficulties and older children with obesity, suggests that the trend towards early weaning should be reversed. Many nutritionists advise the postponement of weaning until six months.

Skimmed milk

This should not be given to children under five years old as it does not provide enough calories and lacks the fat-soluble vitamins. However, semi-skimmed milk can be given to children of two years old and above, provided they are growing well.

BELOW *Growing babies need good nutrition.*

Introducing solid food

The first solid food for a baby usually consists of cooked and puréed fruit and vegetables, or specially prepared baby cereals. It is best to avoid food with added salt or sugar.

When you are preparing a healthy meal for yourself, you can save time by sieving a small portion for the baby, such as avocado flesh.

A baby's appetite will grow as he or she grows, until about one year when growth slows down and the appetite usually decreases. At about this time babies and toddlers often develop likes and dislikes. It is best to avoid battles about food: if you continue to offer nutritious food and avoid giving sweets, you can trust your toddler to eat what he or she needs.

What about food supplements?

Giving supplements to healthy young babies and infants is controversial. Many parents and paediatricians think that breast milk from a well-nourished mother together with well-chosen nutritious solid food is sufficient. Others feel happier with a supplement that provides the recommended levels of minerals and vitamins (see p130–139).

When a supplement is given, it is usual to use a liquid preparation for the first year or so, and then a preparation that can be chewed. It is important to follow the instructions on the bottle: if in doubt, seek professional advice.

To avoid dietary imbalance, mineral and vitamin supplements should not be taken in large doses, except with professional guidance.

Can too much be toxic?

Vitamins A and D can both be toxic, so follow the dosage advice. Avoid high doses of cod liver oil.

RIGHT *During the first year of life growth is rapid and a baby's appetite also increases.*

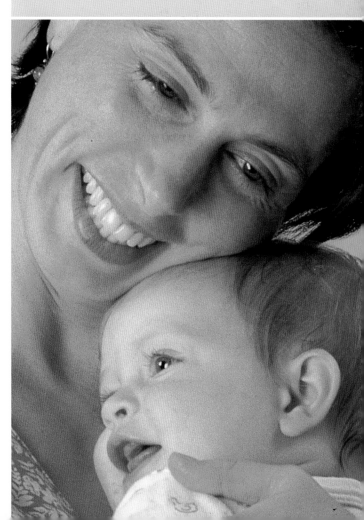

> ### BABY-TIPS
>
> When you prepare your baby's food, freeze one or more baby-sized portions in the container used for ice cubes, for another day.
>
> If you defrost and/or heat your baby's food in a microwave oven, ALWAYS STIR IT, in case heating has been uneven and ALWAYS test the temperature before serving.
>
> Raw vegetables help your baby during teething: let him or her chew on a whole peeled carrot, or a stick of celery or peeled cucumber.

From two to twelve years

Mental development and learning are very rapid between the ages of two and 12 years and good nutrition is essential to enable children to develop their full potential. In addition, physical growth is continuing. Children learn good eating habits from the example set by their parents and a good diet can educate their taste. Snacks and treats should be chosen from wholesome foods such as fruit, popcorn, cheese and raw vegetables, which children often prefer to cooked vegetables. High-fat, high-salt snacks and fizzy drinks should be avoided as far as possible.

YOUR
SPECIAL
NEEDS

Pre-school needs

The slowing of growth that marks the end of the first year continues until the child is about three. Many two-year-olds develop strong likes and dislikes as well as going through phases of eating virtually nothing and, although this makes parents very anxious, it is probably best to avoid battles about food. Simply continue to provide good food and try to avoid offering bribes and rewards in the form of sweet food.

Small children's likes and dislikes can change very rapidly, so it is worth trying again, after a suitable amount of time has passed and the memory forgotten, with a food that has previously been rejected.

LEFT
Encourage children to snack on fresh fruit rather than sweets or crisps.

The early years of school

It is impossible to keep school-aged children away from peer pressure to eat a less nutritious diet. However, encouraging an interest in wholesome food, reaching agreement with them about planning and preparing meals, and enlisting their help in preparing their packed lunches, all help to interest them in good nutrition.

Children perform better at school if they have eaten breakfast, preferably consisting of whole-grain cereals plus a protein food, such as an egg. If breakfast consists of sugary foods, the initial burst of energy will soon wear off.

After-school snacks should be low in refined sugar. Whole-grain foods, nuts and fruit, including dried fruit, are ideal. Although snacks should not be allowed to spoil the appetite for a family meal, a child who is too hungry may not be able to eat either.

ABOVE *Dried fruit provides a healthy and filling after-school snack.*

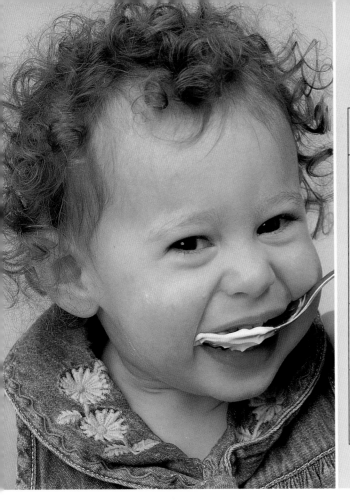

AGE	AVERAGE CALORIE NEEDS PER DAY	AVERAGE PROTEIN NEEDS (G PER DAY)
0–3 months	515–545	12.5g
4–6 months	645–690	12.7–13g
7–9 months	765–825	13.7–14g
10–12 months	865–920	14–14.9g
1–3 years	1,165–1,300-	14.5–16g
4–6 years	1,545–1,800	19.7–24g
7–10 years	1,740–2,000	28–28.3g
BOYS		
11–14 years	2,220–2,500	42.1–45g
15–18 years	2,755–3,000	55.2–59g
GIRLS		
11–14 years	1,845–2,200	41.2–46g
15–18 years	2,110–2,200	44–45g

ABOVE *Try to avoid battles about food.*

Providing for energy and growth

Children need plenty of carbohydrate for energy and protein for growth. The exact amounts depend on how much they weigh and how much they do. Young children may eat very little if they have a minor illness, but make up for it by eating more than usual when they recover. The average figures given above provide a rough guide.

Children will nearly always eat:

• Home-made rissoles or burgers, either vegetarian or meat, with wholemeal buns, and tomato sauce, home-made if possible

• Baked potato with cheddar or cottage cheese, or minced meat, and/or baked beans

• Pizza: use a wholemeal base and add a generous topping that includes acceptable vegetables and cheese

• Pasta, preferably wholemeal, with a sauce made from tomato, cheese or meat

• Whole-flour pancakes (see p20). If you serve them with molasses (see p26) you will be providing a rich mixture of B-vitamins and calcium

What about supplements?

Minerals and vitamins are best obtained from a broadly based whole-food diet. However, many parents provide mineral and vitamin supplements to reassure themselves that their children are obtaining the basic recommended allowances If you are giving supplements, follow the dosage advice on the bottle, as it changes according to age. Vitamins A and D and some minerals, such as selenium, are toxic at relatively low doses.

To avoid dietary imbalance, mineral and vitamin supplements should not usually be taken in large doses.

Adolescence

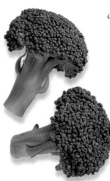

The teenage years can be a difficult time of life. Physical growth and mental development are rapid, boys' voices change, girls start having periods, and most teenagers have to face taking public examinations for the first time. Teenagers develop unusual eating habits and often eat too many fried, fast and junk foods. On the other hand, the reverse can also be true as social pressures can lead them to cut back drastically on food, often without thought to their nutritional needs. Such diets are often deficient in protein, minerals and vitamins, and this can have a negative effect on mood and behaviour, as well as physical health.

Boys

Between the ages of 13 and 18, boys may put on up to 9kg (20lb) and grow up to 12cm (5in) in a year. They need plenty of protein to build the larger muscles that are developing. Very active adolescent boys may consume up to 4,000 calories a day. This is a generous allowance, which should easily provide enough minerals and vitamins, but frequently does not as boys often avoid vegetables and whole-grain carbohydrates.

Girls

Adolescence in girls starts earlier, with the main growth spurt usually occurring between 11 and 16 years. They may grow up to 10cm (4in) in a year and put on up to 8kg (18lb). More weight-conscious than boys, they usually consume fewer calories, and are therefore even more prone to nutritional deficiencies. When their monthly periods start, girls need more iron as well as calcium and zinc. Irregular and painful periods can be caused by nutritional deficiencies and, although the birth-control pill is sometimes prescribed for these problems, it also increases the need for certain nutrients (see p108–109).

Fast food

A daily diet of bread and cheese, sweets and packaged snack foods, washed down with a fizzy drink, will be deficient in minerals, many vitamins and possibly even protein. Equally, meals from fast-food outlets usually contain too much salt, fat, chemical additives, preservatives and

FAR LEFT *Broccoli is a nutritional superstar: eat it raw, or only very lightly cooked to preserve its goodness.*

LEFT *Snack on nuts and seeds rather than sweets or potato crisps.*

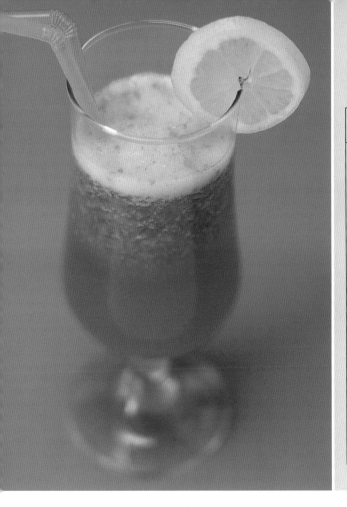

ABOVE *For extra nutritional value, sweeten freshly made fruit drinks with molasses.*

> ### SUPER-CHARGED SNACKS
>
> • Why not try a fresh fruit drink (see p69) and add 1–2 teaspoonfuls of molasses for a real mineral and vitamin boost? Molasses can also be spread on bread.
>
> • Snack on nuts and seeds. Feast on the minerals, protein and good-quality oils that they contain.
>
> • Dried fruits, such as raisins, apricots and dates, are much more nutritious than chocolate.

---

sugar, and insufficient fibre, even though the protein content may be adequate.

Particular needs in adolescence

CALCIUM AND IRON are both needed for growth. VITAMIN D, which is needed to enable the body to absorb calcium, is often deficient if the diet contains no milk. Once a girl's periods have started, her need for iron increases.

CALCIUM, MAGNESIUM, BORON, VITAMINS D AND K, ZINC, COPPER AND MANGANESE are all needed to build strong and healthy bones. PHOSPHORUS is also required but is unlikely to be lacking in the diet. Failure to build good bones may increase the risk of osteoporosis (see p61) in later life.

ZINC, MANGANESE, CHROMIUM AND SELENIUM are often low in the diet of teenagers as they tend to eat too much refined carbohydrate, such as white flour and sugar.

VITAMINS C AND P can be deficient if insufficient fresh fruit and vegetables are eaten.

THE B-VITAMINS can easily fall below the required level in adolescents. This is particularly important for girls taking birth-control pills and teenagers taking antibiotics for acne.

ZINC, VITAMINS A AND F, especially the omega-3 fats (see p51–53), may help the complexion.

Are food supplements necessary?

Supplements should not act as substitutes for a nutritious diet. There are substances in food that we need, but have not yet identified and these are not included in supplements.

To avoid dietary imbalance, mineral and vitamin supplements should not usually be taken in large doses.

Adult life

A healthy and nutritious diet is one that contains sufficient minerals, vitamins, carbohydrate, protein and fat to keep your body healthy through the childbearing years and into old age. However, the pace of adult life can make such a diet very difficult to maintain and supplements can then prove valuable.

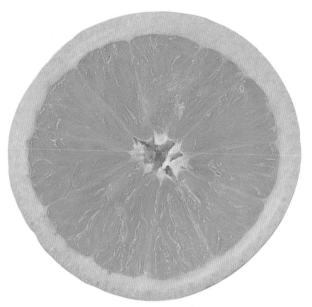

Adult women

Women require fewer calories than men, but they need almost as much protein and more iron during their childbearing years. The calorie restriction that many women impose on themselves can result in a diet deficient in a number of nutrients. If they lack sufficient cholesterol they can develop irregular hormonal cycles, loss of fertility, an early menopause and osteoporosis (see p61). Poor nutrition can also affect the success of pregnancy and women should eat well for several months before planning to become pregnant.

Special needs of women

CALCIUM, IRON AND ZINC are lost in the normal menstrual cycle.

CALCIUM AND MAGNESIUM can help to

LEFT *Citrus fruits provide some of the vitamin C that all adults need.*

reduce period pains (see p62), and together with VITAMINS K AND D, BORON, ZINC, COPPER AND MANGANESE build strong bones (see osteoporosis p61).

VITAMIN C AND THE B-VITAMINS are needed in at least the recommended amounts (see p130–139) to maintain health.

To avoid dietary imbalance, mineral and vitamin supplements should not be taken in large doses, except with professional guidance.

If you take birth-control pills

Women who take the birth-control pill may find that it can alter their nutritional needs, and this can be a problem for growing teenagers. A high-nutrient diet as suggested in the checklist on page 109 is essential. If you are concerned about weight gain, eat proportionately more vegetables than fruit, as they generally contain fewer calories.

The birth-control pill increases the level of copper in the blood and supplements are unnecessary, but if you take a multi-mineral supplement, up to 1mg of copper is safe. Avoid too much iron

ABOVE *Try to eat at least five portions of fresh fruit and vegetables every day*

if your periods are light. The level of vitamin A in the blood increases while birth-control pills are taken. As vitamin A is known to cause damage to the unborn baby, some doctors advise delaying a pregnancy for three months after discontinuing the birth-control pill.

VITAMINS C, E, K AND THE B-VITAMINS, especially **B6 AND FOLIC ACID, BETA-CAROTENE, ZINC AND SELENIUM** all help to counterbalance changes caused by the birth-control pill.

Adult men

Active men usually require more calories than women and, if they wish to become fathers, they should eat a particularly good diet during the four months before the planned time of conception. This may seem a long time, but it takes more than 100 days for the cells in the testicles to undergo the number of cell divisions required to become sperm. At this time smoking and alcohol intake should be reduced or stopped.

Special needs of men

The following nutrients may help to promote an active sex life and successful fatherhood.

VITAMINS A, C, E, F AND FOLIC ACID are needed for sperm production.

CALCIUM, MAGNESIUM, ZINC AND SULPHUR, VITAMINS C AND B12 AND INOSITAL are all present in sperm and may contribute to fertility.

ZINC AND SELENIUM are needed to replace losses in spermatic fluid.

ZINC, MAGNESIUM AND VITAMIN B6 may help if the sex drive has decreased.

To avoid dietary imbalance, mineral and vitamin supplements should not usually be taken in large doses.

RIGHT *Easy-to-prepare meals like tabbouleh (see p87) can provide a rich selection of nutrients.*

CHECKLIST FOR A BALANCED DIET

Adults should aim for:

- A diet that varies from day to day and season to season
- At least five portions of a variety of fresh fruit and vegetables each day (one portion is 100g (3½oz).
- High-fibre carbohydrate food chosen from whole grain products, pulses, fruits and vegetables
- Adequate, but not excessive, protein from animal and vegetable sources
- A moderate intake of fats and oils
- A modest consumption of alcoholic drinks, if desired
- Minimal intake of sugar and other refined carbohydrates, such as white flour
- Avoidance of excessive salt and food additives, such as colourings, flavourings and preservatives

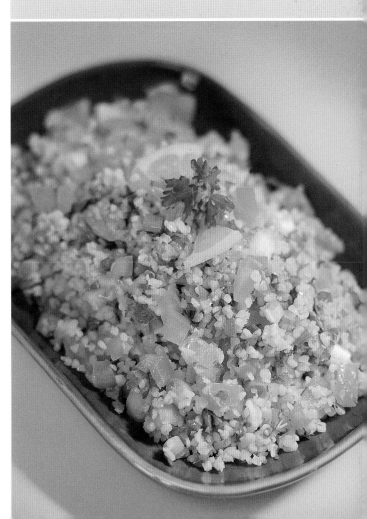

Pregnancy and breast feeding

'Eating for two' while you are pregnant or breast feeding does not mean eating twice as much. You will require up to 200 to 300 extra calories a day during pregnancy, and between 600 and 1,000 extra calories during the later stages of breast feeding. Doctors now usually prescribe a small dose of folic acid during the first three months of pregnancy, and iron supplements later in pregnancy. You should seek professional advice if you wish to take any other mineral, vitamin or herbal supplements during this period.

YOUR
SPECIAL
NEEDS

What should I eat?

Continue the healthy diet suggested on p109, but you will need extra supplies of protein to build the baby's tissues and the placenta. This can be decreased a little when you are breast feeding, but you still need more protein than usual. Ensure that you eat food containing sufficient minerals and vitamins. If your diet is inadequate, those nutrients needed by the baby will be taken from your tissues and bones, and can create a deficit.

What foods should be avoided?

Avoid refined carbohydrates, artificial flavourings, colourings and preservatives. Keep tea, coffee and alcoholic drinks to a minimum and try to stop smoking. Avoid liver, which can contain a large amount of vitamin A (see p43), and soft cheeses and pâté, which can contain listeria. Listeria is a cause of miscarriage and stillbirth and, unlike most bacteria, grows at refrigerator temperatures. If you eat pre-cooked foods, they should be heated thoroughly to kill any listeria.

Baby boosters

The following list indicates particular ways in which minerals and vitamins provide for your needs and those of your baby during pregnancy and while you are breast feeding.

CALCIUM AND MAGNESIUM are needed for the baby's teeth and bones, muscle action (including the heart), blood clotting and nervous system. They also help to counteract high blood pressure in the mother, and can help reduce muscle cramps, insomnia, varicose veins and haemorrhoids (piles).

IRON is essential for the blood cells

RIGHT *You will need folic acid and iron supplements during pregnancy.*

LEFT *Eat a dry biscuit before getting up in the morning to relieve nausea.*

of both mother and baby. In addition to any iron supplement prescribed by your doctor, eat iron-rich food. Iron is absorbed best when food rich in vitamin C is eaten at the same time.

ZINC aids normal development of the baby's immune system, and may help to counter-act stretch marks and insomnia in the mother.

SODIUM is needed in greater amounts during pregnancy. Too little may cause damage to the placenta and may also cause pregnant women to crave pickles, olives or sauerkraut. Too much sodium may lead to water retention and raised blood pressure. To achieve a balance, listen to your body's needs and seek advice.

IODINE needs are increased during pregnancy and it is best obtained from sea salt, sea fish and sea vegetables such as kelp, rather than iodized salt which sometimes contains other chemicals that are less welcome.

FOLIC ACID intake needs are doubled in preg-nancy and deficiency is now known to contribute to spina bifida and other nervous system defects in the baby. Eat plenty of food rich in folic acid as well as taking a prescribed supplement.

VITAMINS A (AS BETA-CAROTENE), C, P, B6 AND E are all needed in increased amounts. Rubbing vitamin E oil into your skin may reduce stretch marks. Vitamins C and P may help to prevent haemorrhoids and varicose veins.

To avoid dietary imbalance, mineral and vitamin supplements should not usually be taken in large doses. except with professional guidance.

RIGHT *Ensure that your diet in preg-nancy provides the extra vitamins and minerals that you and your baby need.*

MORNING SICKNESS

The unpleasant nausea and vomiting that can occur in the morning during the first weeks of pregnancy may be reduced by:

• Avoiding fatty food, sugar, refined white flour, citrus fruits and juice

• Eating small meals frequently and not eating late at night

• Having an early morning snack before getting up (dry biscuits, live yoghurt, soy bean soup or miso [soy bean paste] in hot water)

• Avoiding constipation by eating a diet rich in fibre

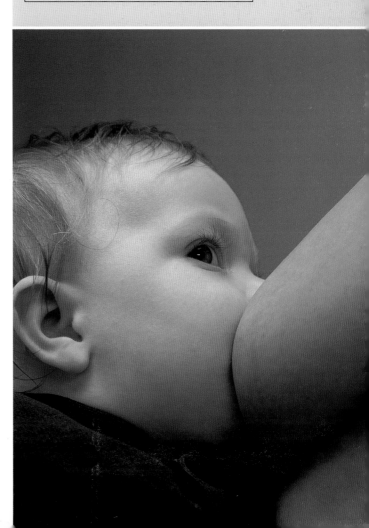

From fifty to sixty-five

Some people love their work and want to continue for as long as possible. Others look forward to the freedom of retirement after many years of work. Whatever the aim, many people in their fifties begin to worry about being fit enough to achieve it. There is growing evidence that many of the diseases and discomforts of old age may be the result of nutritional deficiencies. Although we should probably begin to eat for a healthy old age in our twenties, it is never too late to start.

YOUR
SPECIAL
NEEDS

Staying healthy

We have all met 60-year-olds who seem old, and sprightly 90-year-olds, who seem young. To some extent, of course, this depends on the genes that we have inherited, but getting older is also a state of mind. It is important to have interests outside the home and to engage in regular exercise.

Basic dietary needs do not suddenly change from the balanced diet needed in adult life (see p109). However, energy levels gradually decline and fewer calories are needed. Because of this, you should make every calorie count by avoiding 'empty' calories like white sugar that contain no vitamins or minerals.

Osteoporosis

This bone condition is more common in women. Preventive action can help to prevent fractures in later life (see p61).

Are food supplements needed?

A good diet should supply all the necessary nutrients, but you may wish to take a well-balanced multi-mineral and vitamin supplement anyway. To avoid dietary imbalance, mineral and vitamin supplements should not be taken in large doses, except with professional guidance.

The menopause

Some women hardly notice their menopause, but for many the cessation of their periods is accom-

ABOVE *Kiwi fruit is stuffed with vitamin C, and also contains fibre and potassium.*

LEFT *Some diseases of old age are less likely to occur if you eat a nutrient-rich diet.*

panied by irritability, memory lapses and loss of purpose. Physically, hot flushes, sleep disturbance, weight gain and loss of sex drive can also cause considerable distress.

Action plan for the menopause

Continue to eat the best possible diet (see Adult life, p108–109) so that you are not battling against nutritional deficiencies.

● For hot flushes consider taking **VITAMIN E AND SELENIUM** (but see individual sections for cautions). They seem to work together to control the problems of temperature regulation that occur with decreased output of female hormones. **BORON** may also help (see p64) and may protect against osteoporosis (see p61). **VITAMINS C AND P** strengthen the blood vessel and capillary walls and can reduce flushing. Regular exercise, including an active sex life, helps to mobilize some of the oestrogen that is stored in fatty tissues. Try to avoid large meals, alcohol and caffeine as they tend to dilate the small blood vessels in the skin.

● For insomnia, **MAGNESIUM AND CALCIUM** at bedtime can be helpful, as can sedative herbs taken as teas (such as chamomilla, limeflower or fennel), or in tablet form. Regular outdoor exercise may improve sleep and strengthen the bones.

● For vaginal dryness, local application of **VITAMIN E** can help. It can be obtained by puncturing a vitamin E capsule and squeezing out the contents. If the lining of the vagina has become cracked and damaged, calendula cream may be applied to speed healing.

IGHT A drink f milk at edtime can be elaxing and romote sleep.

AR RIGHT Whole rains and seeds are ich in minerals nd vitamin E.

> ### WHAT ABOUT HORMONE REPLACEMENT THERAPY (HRT)?
>
> Many women, in consultation with their doctors, find that HRT is the ideal approach to menopause. If you do take it you should follow the dietary advice given for the birth-control pill on p108–109. Unfortunately, if you are one of the 40–85 per cent of women who would have developed hot flushes, HRT only postpones these symptoms. Currently, there is great interest in relieving menopausal symptoms with the many plants that contain oestrogen-like substances and natural progesterone, but this approach needs further scientific evaluation. Remember that herbs can be very powerful and you should seek professional advice before taking them.

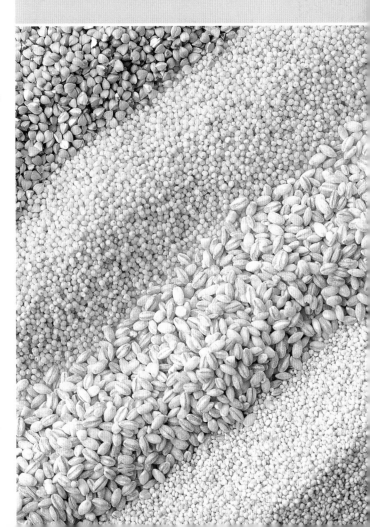

The over sixty-fives

Malnutrition is common in older people. This may be the result of poor digestion, problems with the teeth and chewing, or simply insufficient energy to shop and cook. There is growing evidence that good nutrition can help older people to remain independent, alert and healthy, but dietary changes should be introduced gradually so that the digestion has time to adapt.

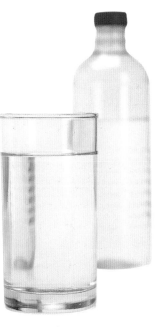

LEFT *Drink plenty of water for a healthy skin and to help your digestive system.*

Adding life to years

Slowing down the ageing process is less a question of adding years to life than of adding life and wellbeing to the years of living. To achieve this:

- Eat regularly. Many older people do not obtain enough calories. If your appetite is small, try to eat little and often.
- Eat fresh foods. If you find it difficult to chew fruit and vegetables, use a food processor, liquidizer or juicer.
- Eat whole grains. These are full of minerals and help to prevent constipation.
- Drink plenty of water. This helps to avoid constipation and keeps the skin healthy.
- Watch your weight. Being 2.5–5kg (5–10lb) overweight is healthier than being underweight.

LEFT *A drink of vegetable juice is rich in vitamins and minerals.*

Making life easier

Preparing food takes time and energy: prepare two or three meals at the same time and store the extra ones in the refrigerator or freezer.

Share meals with friends and take turns to cook, but agree to keep the meals simple.

Try to avoid 'empty calories', such as refined sugar, which will spoil the appetite without providing any minerals or vitamins.

Instead of a cup of tea or coffee and a biscuit mid-morning, have a fruit drink (see p69), or fresh vegetable juice. These can easily contain 170–220g (6–8oz) of fruit or vegetables rich in minerals and vitamins.

Take moderate exercise, preferably out of doors, as often as possible. This will keep your bones strong and stimulate your appetite.

Special needs

For older people, the daily nutrient recommendations are relatively meaningless as the bodily processes become less efficient. However, ensuring a good supply of vitamins and minerals can only be helpful and many nutritionists routinely recommend a regular, well-balanced mineral and vitamin supplement.

VITAMIN A keeps your skin, eyesight and immune system healthy. Avoid too much retinol: beta-carotene is safer (see p41–44).

VITAMINS B1, B2, B6, B12 AND COPPER help to maintain energy levels.

FOLIC ACID AND VITAMIN B12 prevent anaemia. **IRON** is also needed, but high doses should be avoided (see p72–73).

ZINC helps to fight infections, and promote healing. It may also inhibit cancer.

CALCIUM, MAGNESIUM, BORON, VITAMINS D AND K, ZINC, COPPER AND MANGANESE are all needed to maintain strong and healthy bones. **PHOSPHORUS** is also needed but is unlikely to be deficient in the diet.

CHROMIUM keeps the amount of sugar in the blood at the correct level. It can be taken as brewer's yeast or commercially prepared glucose tolerance factor (see GTF p85).

SODIUM AND POTASSIUM can become unbalanced in older people. This can usually be remedied by decreasing the amount of salt in the diet and eating plenty of fruit and vegetables.

VITAMIN E, SELENIUM, MANGANESE AND COPPER help to rid the body of free radicals that can cause tissue damage.

VITAMIN C AND P help to reduce infection, protect against the formation of cataracts and, possibly, to inhibit cancer. They keep the blood vessels strong and help to control the level of fats in the blood.

VITAMIN F can reduce the risk of heart disease.

To avoid dietary imbalance, mineral and vitamin supplements should not be taken in large doses, except with professional guidance.

RIGHT *Vitamin A helps to keep your skin healthy and your eyesight and immune system in working order.*

HERBAL HELPERS

GARLIC helps to fight infection and may reduce the risk of heart disease (see caution on p93)

CAYENNE CHILLI stimulates energy and the circulation without raising blood pressure. It may also help to keep the bowel regular (see caution on p94).

Always follow the manufacturer's instructions when available.

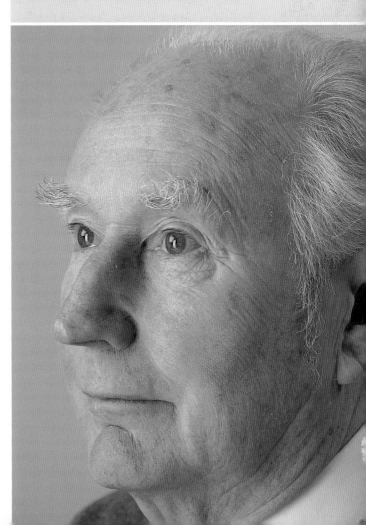

Injuries and surgery

Whenever the skin is broken or cut either through an accident or for medical reasons, harmful bacteria gain access to the underlying tissues. The conditions in the wound are ideal for bacteria to reproduce. It is warm and moist, there is a plentiful supply of protein and, if the wound is dressed, it is also dark. A wound infection can develop very quickly and this can slow down the healing process and may eventually overwhelm the immune system. It is possible, however, to build up your defences against this happening through your diet or with supplements.

YOUR
SPECIAL
NEEDS

Before an operation

About three or four weeks before the operation, in addition to your normal healthy diet, it may be advisable to:

• Eat plenty of good-quality protein to ensure that the body is able to heal damaged tissue without delay

• Eat high-fibre foods and yoghurt to replenish the natural, helpful bacteria that live benignly in the intestine

• Consume plenty of calcium as it is needed to regulate many of the cells' activities. Ideally, the calcium should come from a variety of sources including greens, grains and nuts

• Eat foods that contain vitamin F

• Avoid stimulants, such as coffee, drugs and all types of tobacco

• A few days before the operation, eat plenty of fruit, vegetables and juices, less protein and fewer starchy foods than usual

• You may wish to take extra minerals and vitamins for two to three weeks before an operation and four to six weeks afterwards

After an operation or injury

After surgery or an injury, the body has several tasks. It has to repair tissue damage and recover from any anaesthetic, either local or general, and any other necessary drugs e.g. for pain relief. Finally, the shock and stress of events can alter normal body function, and recovery from this may increase the body's need of nutrients.

Hospital food can often be less than satisfactory and, if you are used to eating whole foods that are largely chemical-free and a good supply of fruit and vegetables, it may differ considerably from your usual diet.

With the agreement of your surgeon, you could ask your relatives to bring in fresh fruits and vegetables, take high-protein powders to speed the repair of your tissues, and mineral and vitamin supplements.

FAR LEFT Grapes are a popular choice because they are easily digested during convalescence.

BELOW Orange juice or other sources of vitamin C should be taken several times a day.

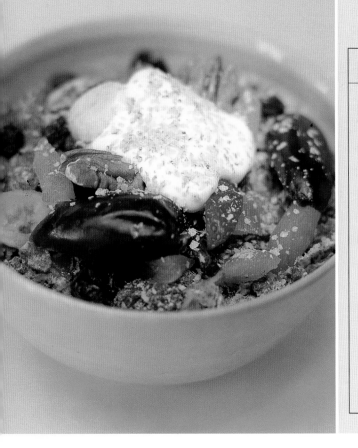

HERBAL HELPERS

HORSETAIL is high in silica, which is a mineral that strengthens tissues (see caution on p95).

GOLDENSEAL helps to ward off infection (see caution on p96).

Always follow the manufacturer's instructions when available.

The healers

VITAMIN A boosts the immune system and helps in the repair of tissues, and BETA-CAROTENE supplies extra vitamin A, if needed, and also acts as an anti-oxidant.

VITAMINS C AND P aid the repair of tissues, and should be taken in several doses each day as they are quickly lost in the urine.

ZINC is a great healer and enables the body to ward off any infection as well as being essential in the repair of damaged tissues.

MAGNESIUM activates many of the biochemical processes of healing.

The B-VITAMINS are all needed for the normal supply of energy, and an effective nervous system. In particular, vitamin B2 is needed for tissue repair and vitamin B5 for its anti-stress function.

VITAMIN K enables the blood to clot, and allows the early stages of scab and scar formation to proceed.

SELENIUM, COPPER, IRON, CALCIUM, POTASSIUM, MANGANESE, MOLYBDENUM AND COBALT all have a role in the healing process. In particular, iron is needed if there has been blood loss.

VITAMINS C, A, SELENIUM AND ZINC are the main nutrients needed to overcome the effects of an anaesthetic and other medication.

VITAMIN F aids wound healing.

VITAMIN E act as an anti-oxidant, but should not be taken in large doses as it can interfere with blood clotting.

To avoid dietary imbalance, mineral, and vitamin supplements should not be taken in large doses, except with professional guidance.

Fighting infection and cancer

The immune system acts in a wide variety of ways to protect the body from infection, and the formation of cancers. If you are abnormally tired, catch frequent colds or other infections, your immune system may not be working as effectively as it could be. It may be overloaded or undernourished, especially if it is dealing with a long-term allergic condition. Try nurturing your immune system with a little loving care. You may be surprised at the result.

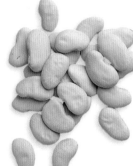

LEFT
Cooked, dried butterbeans are a rich source of fibre.

Lightening the load

We are all exposed to industrial or other man-made chemicals in the atmosphere, in food and often at work. It is part of the function of the immune system to detoxify these harmful chemicals.

The first step is to reduce the load on your immune system by avoiding exposure to unnecessary chemicals. Restricting alcohol intake, giving up smoking and avoiding smoky rooms can all help. Other recreational drugs should be avoided and pharmaceutical drugs taken sparingly or not at all, if possible. If you are exposed to industrial chemicals, follow carefully any instructions given for your protection.

You can reduce your consumption of food additives by avoiding foods that contain preservatives, colouring agents and flavourings. It is a good idea to minimize the amount of smoked, salted, pickled or barbecued food that you eat. It may help to eat organic produce when possible, and to drink filtered or spring water.

Try to reduce the stress in your life. Make time for regular relaxation and enjoyment and don't deprive yourself of sleep. Always try to take your full holiday entitlement.

If you do not take any exercise, try to set aside some time to devote to it. At the very least, go for a walk or a cycle ride every weekend, building up to two, then three times a week. Regular exercise directly benefits the immune system and keeps it working effectively.

If you suffer from an allergy, it may be acting as a depressant on your immune system. Try to reduce this effect by avoiding the cause, seeking homeopathic treatment, or consulting a nutritional or allergy practitioner for advice on how to overcome it.

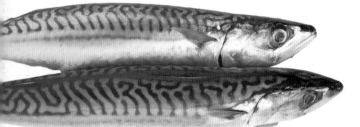

LEFT *If possible, eat oily fish once or twice a week.*

Immunity enhancers

The immune system is best nourished by eating a good-quality diet and drinking plenty of water. This means eating lots of fresh fruit and vegetables, a reasonable quantity of meat and fish, and very little sugar and fat.

If you are a vegetarian, try to eat a wide variety of protein-rich foods. A high-fibre diet appears to reduce the risk of bowel cancer. It is also a good idea to try to maintain your weight at the correct level for your height and age, as some cancers are known to be more common in over-weight people.

The following nutrients may be of particular benefit.

MAGNESIUM, ZINC AND THE B-VITAMINS, ESPECIALLY B6, PANTOTHENIC ACID AND FOLIC ACID: these nutrients help the human body to maintain the immune system in a healthy working state.

ANTI-OXIDANT MINERALS AND VITAMINS, SUCH AS ZINC, SELENIUM, VITAMINS C, E AND P, AND BETA-CAROTENE: these help to neutralize the unstable substances, known as free radicals, that can damage cells.

VITAMIN F and other good-quality oils and fat from vegetable sources (preferably cold-pressed), and oily fish may also be beneficial.

Excessive animal fat may suppress immunity and appear to increase the risk of breast, bowel and prostate cancers. Some nutritionists recommend restricting all fat to less than 50g (1¼oz) a day but, if you do this, make sure that you are still getting sufficient fat-soluble vitamins (A, D, E and K).

To avoid dietary imbalance, mineral and vitamin supplements should not be taken in large doses, except with professional guidance.

RIGHT *Reduce the stress in your life by practising relaxation techniques.*

CONSIDER TAKING
ONE OF THE FOLLOWING
HERBAL HELPERS

GARLIC helps to fight infection and may stimulate the immune system in other ways (see p93 for caution).

LIQUORICE stimulates the adrenal gland, counteracting stress, inflammation and infection (see p97 for caution).

ECHINACEA has been used to fight various infections (see p95 for caution).

GOLDENSEAL can help to overcome bacterial infection and parasitic invasion (see p96 for caution).

Always follow the manufacturer's instructions.

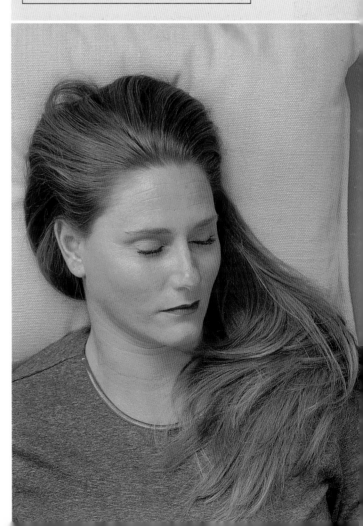

Preventing heart disease

The twentieth century has seen an unprecedented epidemic of heart disease in the developed world. People from other cultures are also affected when they move into developed countries, and it has even begun to affect parts of the Third World where people have copied the unhealthily sedentary, junk-food oriented lifestyles of the West. We do not yet fully understand what has gone wrong, but we have at last begun to investigate and tackle the problem.

Known risks

- Tobacco smoking is the single most easily avoidable cause of heart disease.
- Raised cholesterol levels in the blood undoubtedly increase the risk of heart disease. It is likely, however, that dietary deficiencies also contribute to the narrowing of arteries in the heart muscle that can cause angina and, if they become totally blocked, heart attacks.
- Hypertension is the technical term for raised blood pressure. It has many causes and can itself cause heart attacks, heart failure (when the heart becomes less effective) and strokes.

- Obesity can contribute to raised blood pressure, diabetes and raised cholesterol, as well as reduce the inclination to exercise.
- Stress can also lead to raised blood pressure through increased adrenaline (epinephrine) output, and its effects may be intensified through excessive amounts of caffeine, alcohol and an unbalanced diet.
- Lack of exercise means that the heart muscle does not get a 'work out', which it needs, like other muscles of the body, to remain strong.
- Drinking soft water can mean an inadequate intake of magnesium and calcium.
- Family history cannot, of course, be changed. Heart disease does 'run' in some families, but it is not inevitable, and members of such families may well avoid it by adopting a healthy lifestyle.

Checklist to a healthy heart

- Stop smoking.
- If you are overweight, try to reduce your weight to within about 10 per cent of the ideal weight for your height.

ABOVE *Garlic helps to normalize the level of fat in the blood.*

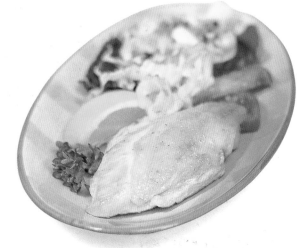

LEFT *Try to reduce the amount of fat in your diet to around 55–80g (2–3oz) a day.*

- Eat more fruit, vegetables and whole grains: the fibre that these contain helps to reduce cholesterol levels. Eat nuts and seeds in moderation.
- Reduce intake of animal fat both in red meats, cheese, butter and dripping, and in cakes, pastries and pies. Try to reduce the fat in your diet to about 25–30 per cent of your total calorie intake (around 55–80g (2–3oz) per day.
- Eat fish, especially oily fish, at least twice a week.
- Limit your intake of salt, sugar and alcohol.
- Take regular exercise three or four times a week. (Consult your doctor before starting vigorous exercise if you are over 30, or have any medical condition.)

Help your heart to health

MAGNESIUM may be the single most important nutrient to protect against heart disease, so eating food that is rich in magnesium should be a high priority. It helps to dilate the arteries of the heart, steadies the activity of the heart muscle, and has a generally mild tranquillizing action.

SELENIUM AND VITAMIN E are antioxidants that are thought to be able to reduce the risk of heart attacks.

ZINC helps to repair damaged tissues, but in high doses (over 100mg a day) may increase cholesterol levels.

CALCIUM works with magnesium to keep the heart beating normally.

VITAMINS C, E, B3, B6, F, CHROMIUM AND SELENIUM all help to prevent the fatty deposits (atheroma) that cause narrowing of the arteries carrying oxygen to the heart muscle.

To avoid dietary imbalance, mineral and vitamin supplements should not be taken in large doses, except with professional guidance.

RIGHT *Maintain the strength of your heart muscle by taking regular (and frequent!) exercise.*

CONSIDER TAKING ONE OF THE FOLLOWING HERBAL HELPERS:

GARLIC helps to normalize the level of fat in the blood and can reduce the risk of blood clots forming in the arteries (see p93 for caution).

CAYENNE CHILLI may reduce the risk of blood clots in the arteries (see p94 for caution).

GINGER can stimulate the circulation (see p99 for caution).

OATS can help to reduce the level of cholesterol in the blood (see p94 for caution).

Always follow the manufacturer's instructions when available.

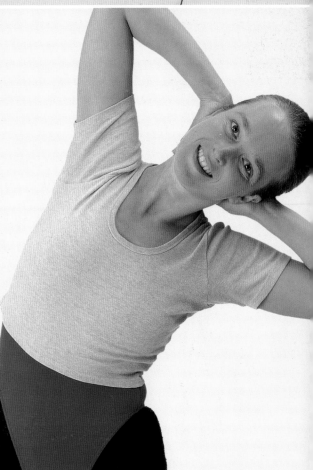

Active living

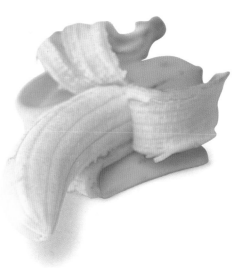

If you wish to train for competitive sport or simply to keep fit, you can do much to maximize the effort you put into your exercise routine by paying attention to your diet and avoiding the pitfalls of dehydration. Intense, strenuous exercise appears to increase the body's need for anti-oxidant minerals and vitamins. These nutrients will help to reduce soreness after exercise and minimize damage to tissues and joints that can be caused by free radicals.

Keeping the food balance right

When you undertake serious training or take regular prolonged exercise, around 50–60 per cent of your calorie intake should come from carbohydrate, at least half of which should be whole grains, pulses and starchy vegetables. Up to another 25 per cent of calories should come from good-quality protein, and between 15 and 30 per cent from fat. For a 3,000kcal diet this would mean 50–100g (2–3oz) of fat, much of which should come from vegetable sources, such as olives, avocados, seeds, nuts, and oily fish.

Maintaining your energy

The body stores carbohydrate as glycogen in the muscles and liver. These stores are increased by regular training and by a diet rich in carbohydrate. Glycogen provides energy by being broken down into glucose, and is also needed to release energy stored in the body's fat. As you use up these stores, your body temperature rises and you start to sweat. If the lost fluid is not replaced, your performance will deteriorate.

Sports drinks

Loss of fluid through perspiration is best replaced by drinking water. Water containing small amounts of sugar and sodium is absorbed into the body more quickly, but too much salt and/or sugar slows water absorption, and discomfort may occur.

You can make your own isotonic drinks by diluting one part of fruit juice with one part of water, or one part of fruit squash with four parts of water, and adding 1–1.5g of salt to each litre. Some commercial sports drinks contain glucose polymers, which may be helpful if you exercise vigorously for more than 90 minutes. Avoid caffeine as it increases your fluid loss (as urine) and can cause anxiety and/or a rapid heart beat.

ABOVE *Bananas are bursting with potassium as well as containing other valuable minerals and vitamins.*

LEFT *Olives are not only full of health-giving oil but also contain many valuable minerals and vitamins.*

Sporting needs

Supplements containing 100–200 per cent of the daily recommended intake may be useful, especially mineral supplements as many of these are lost in sweat. However, excessive supplementation will not enhance performance further, and may lead to nutritional imbalance.

SODIUM AND POTASSIUM are needed in correct balance to control the distribution of fluid within the cells of the body, in the tissues between the cells, and in the circulation. They enhance muscle action and prevent spasm, and are both lost in sweat.

CALCIUM AND MAGNESIUM help muscles to contract and relax efficiently, and are essential for strong bones. Magnesium is lost through the skin in sweat, so you need plenty of food rich in magnesium if you take regular exercise.

IRON is needed to replace the red blood cells that are lost by being physically damaged during exercise. It is especially important for women of childbearing age because iron deficiency leads to loss of energy and poor endurance.

CHROMIUM helps the body to regulate the level of sugar in the blood and is lost in the urine more quickly during exercise.

SILICON is needed for tissue flexibility. **VITAMIN C** keeps the connective tissue strong and may reduce the effects of injury. The **B-VITAMINS** are lost more rapidly during exercise. **VITAMIN A, BETA-CAROTENE, VITAMIN E AND SELENIUM** help to reduce tissue damage during exercise and to maintain performance.

To avoid dietary imbalance, mineral and vitamin supplements should not usually be taken in large doses, except with professional guidance.

ABOVE *Seeds are high-protein foods that are also rich in oils and minerals.*

RIGHT *The fluid lost in sweat is best replaced by drinking water.*

IMPROVING YOUR STAMINA

- Minimize fluid loss by drinking before, during and after exercise, especially in warm weather

- Take a snack two hours before training and refuel your glycogen stores with a carbohydrate meal after training

- Increase your glycogen stores by gradually eating more carbohydrate during the week before a big event, but this should not be done more than four times a year

- Avoid sudden weight changes: if you need to gain or lose weight, take your time and only alter your weight by approximately 0.5–1kg (1–2lb) a week

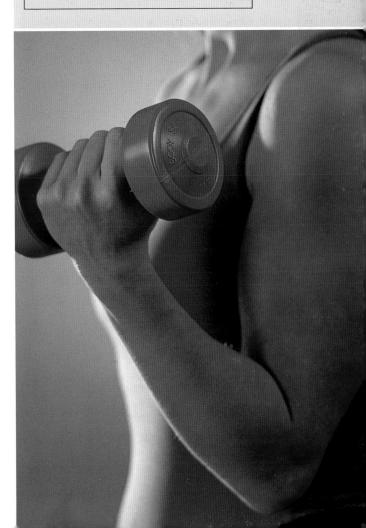

Protection against stress

Although stress is sometimes regarded as a new phenomenon that is peculiar to the late twentieth century, it is likely that human life has always been stressful. In the past, pressures such as simply getting enough to eat, keeping warm, looking after your family, coping with natural disasters and predatory animals all contributed to the stress of daily life.

YOUR
SPECIAL
NEEDS

ABOVE *Avoid the fat in biscuits and chocolate by taking healthy snacks to work.*

The stress response

A modern problem is undoubtedly the sedentary lifestyle that means the extra hormones, particularly adrenaline (epinephrine) and cortisone, which are produced by the body in times of stress and used up by the muscles during exercise, remain in circulation. Symptoms include headache, backache, indigestion, altered bowel and bladder action, palpitations, sighing and air hunger. The immune system is impaired and illnesses such as infection, heart disease and, possibly, cancer, can result. When stressed, the body uses up nutrients more quickly, so increased amounts are needed. The body also produces more free radicals. These are the unstable substances that can cause tissue damage, but can be neutralized if sufficient antioxidant minerals and vitamins are present.

An eating plan for stressful times

Food is, of course, the fuel that keeps you going, but heavy meals can also slow you down. Foods commonly regarded as stimulants, such as coffee, alcohol and sugary snacks, can cause wide fluctua-

tion in blood-sugar levels. This can result in a complete slump just when you want to be alert and clear thinking. Skipped meals can result in poor nutritional intake and lead to illness.

These problems can be avoided if you top up your energy with frequent nutritious snacks by:
- Keeping a supply of seeds and nuts to hand
- Avoiding biscuits, cakes and chocolate and taking healthy snacks to work, such as fruit, celery, carrot or other salad vegetables
- Choosing small portions of food that are low in fat and sugar when you have time for a full meal
- Drinking water frequently as thirst can make you feel hungry when you are not

The business traveller

Gone are the days when business executives could spend several days travelling and arrive already adapted to a new time zone. Flying causes a sudden disruption to body rhythms, as well as exposing the traveller to ozone and radiation at high altitudes, very dry and imperfectly scrubbed and recycled air, and food that is not always very nutritious or appetizing.

The effects of these stresses can be minimized if you keep to the eating plan suggested on p124, drink plenty of water and take extra vitamin C and B-vitamins. If you are prone to constipation, it can be helpful to take a mild laxative as a preventive instead of waiting until you are uncomfortable. Moderate exercise, a sauna and a massage can all help you to relax and adjust to the new time zone.

The stress busters

VITAMIN C is needed in greater amounts during stressful times, and should be taken several times each day as it is lost in the urine.

THE B-VITAMINS are all needed in greater amounts, ideally taken at several meals or snacks. Vitamin B5 is particularly important for the adrenal glands.

VITAMINS A, E, BETA-CAROTENE, ZINC, SELENIUM, COPPER AND MANGANESE are the major anti-oxidant nutrients needed to neutralize free radicals.

POTASSIUM, MAGNESIUM AND CALCIUM all help the body's response to the stress hormones. They help to relax muscles and maintain the normal rhythm of the heart.

CHROMIUM can help to overcome sugar cravings, and thus helps to avoid snacking on nutritionally poor sugary foods (see Glucose Tolerance Factor, p85).

To avoid dietary imbalance, mineral and vitamin supplements should not be taken in large doses, except with professional guidance.

RIGHT A massage can help you to adjust to a new time zone.

HERBAL HELPERS

LIQUORICE has a soothing action which may help at times of stress (see caution on p97)

RELAXING HERBS, such as those found in various herbal teas, can be used to encourage restful sleep.

Always follow the manufacturer's instructions when available.

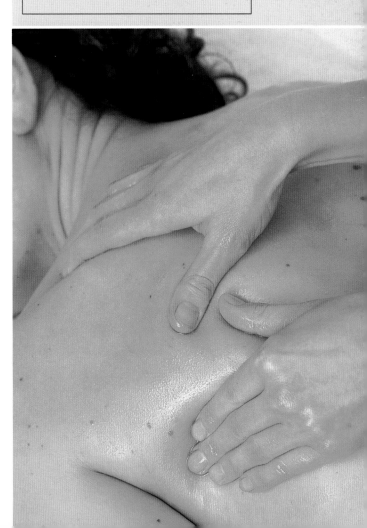

Vegetarians and vegans

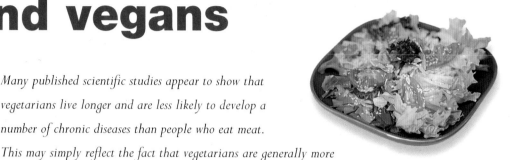

Many published scientific studies appear to show that vegetarians live longer and are less likely to develop a number of chronic diseases than people who eat meat. This may simply reflect the fact that vegetarians are generally more health-conscious. (Some vegetarians, however, especially teenagers, eat grossly inadequate diets.) Everyone would probably benefit from being a vegetarian for at least one or two days a week.

What is a vegetarian?

A vegetarian does not eat meat, fish or poultry. Vegans, in addition, do not drink milk or eat dairy products or eggs either. They may also avoid honey and honey-based products.

Getting the balance right

The ideal and nutritionally rich vegetarian diet is based on a wide range of whole grains, pulses, vegetables, fruits, nuts and seeds, supplemented by dairy produce and eggs if you are not a vegan. Protein deficiency is a common source of anxiety, but an adult with a healthy digestive system may need no more than 50g (2oz) of protein a day. Extra protein is required at times of stress, during adolescence or pregnancy, when breast-feeding, and by athletes and others who lead very active lives. Protein is present in seeds, grains, pulses and nuts but is usually incomplete in these foods. This means that one or more of the amino acids that cannot be produced in our bodies is absent. To overcome this problem, it is important to obtain protein from more than one of these food types, or from eggs, milk and milk products in which the protein is complete. Although not necessary to eat complete protein at every meal, it is wise to have animal protein or vegetable protein from more than one food type each day.

Minerals such as zinc, iron and copper can be deficient if you eat no animal products at all, but the body may adapt and absorb these minerals more efficiently. Calcium deficiency is not as common as might be expected in those who eat a milk-free diet, provided the diet is well-balanced along the lines of the quick guide (see p127).

What about vegans?

Obtaining **VITAMIN B12** can be a problem for vegans, and nutritionists suggest that supplements of this vitamin should be taken at least intermittently to build up stores.

ABOVE *Add vitamin-rich seeds like sunflower and pumpkin seeds to green salads for extra nutrition.*

LEFT *Vegetable juices are rich in minerals, including calcium, but lack fibre.*

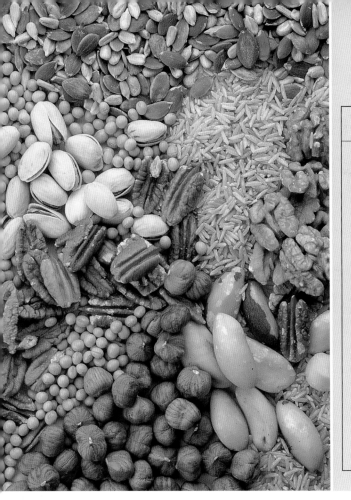

ABOVE *Nuts, grains and seeds are good sources of protein.*

IF BEANS GIVE YOU 'WIND'

Try 'sprouting' beans for a few days before cooking (see p35), or remove outer coverings after soaking overnight. Always cook beans in fresh water (not the water used to soak them in) and boil them briskly for 10 minutes in an uncovered pan before simmering gently until they are soft.

RIGHT *Beans are low in fat and rich in minerals and protein as well as fibre.*

IODINE deficiency has recently been reported in vegans in the United Kingdom where there is no compulsory addition of iodine to food.

It is difficult to obtain adequate nutrition from a vegan diet without mineral (zinc, iron, copper) and vitamin (B12, A and D) supplements during childhood, the teenage years, pregnancy, when breast feeding, and by people with small appetites.

A quick guide for healthy vegetarians and vegans

• Avoid refined foods low in minerals and vitamins, such as white flour and white sugar
• Eat a range of protein-rich foods
• Avoid foods that block the absorption of minerals like calcium, magnesium and zinc. These include bran, and unleavened wheat products, such as chapatis, pastry and biscuits, especially when made with wholemeal flour
• Do not drink tea or coffee at mealtimes
• Eat at least five portions of fresh fruit and vegetables each day
• Remember that people's needs vary considerably, and some people really do need to eat at least some animal protein. This can be indicated if they are constantly tired or lose weight

Supplements as an insurance

A vegetarian formulation of minerals and vitamins, can be taken as a general health insurance measure. For special needs, you should consult the other sections in this chapter.

To avoid dietary imbalance, mineral and vitamin supplements should not be taken in large doses, except with professional guidance.

Healthy skin and hair

Your skin, hair and nails continue to grow throughout your life. They can act as barometers, as they reflect the quality of nourishment that you are giving to your body as a whole, and your general state of physical health. A good diet with plenty of water is one of best ways to improve your appearance, as well as protecting it from the effects of harmful substances.

Looking good

Your skin is the largest organ of your body. It needs a plentiful supply of nutrients because the outer layers, which are constantly being shed, have to be replaced by the division of the deeper cells. Some of these cells are specialized, and divide to form hair and nails.

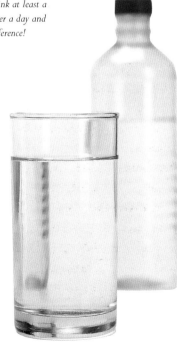

BELOW *Drink at least a litre of water a day and feel the difference!*

Healthy skin is able to provide an effective barrier against the weather and infection. Keeping your skin scrupulously clean helps to banish any harmful bacteria that may be present on the surface of the skin.

Doctors and nutritional therapists may ask for an analysis of the minerals in your hair when they want to judge how good your recent diet has been. They may also examine the nails for evidence of poor nutrition. For example, iron or zinc deficiency can be diagnosed from the appearance of the nails (spoon-shaped nails indicate iron deficiency; white spots indicate zinc deficiency).

Beauty from the inside

A generous intake of fruit and vegetables contains the variety of minerals and vitamins needed to keep your skin, hair and nails healthy. Whole-grain foods, seeds and nuts provide essential fats. The roughage in all these foods, together with at least a litre of water a day, helps to keep the bowel active and the skin clear. Protein is needed for the cells that are dividing in the deeper layers of skin.

ABOVE *Creams that contain vitamin E can help to minimize the formation of scars.*

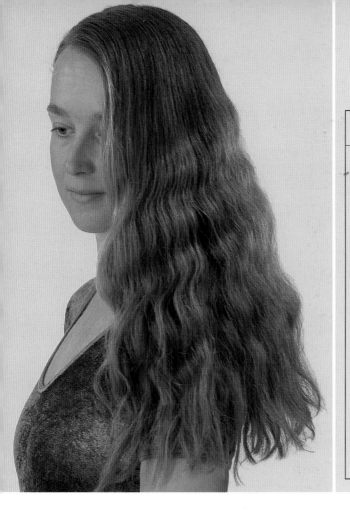

EVERYDAY SKINCARE

SLEEP During good-quality sleep, the body replenishes the skin that has been shed.

SAUNAS Up to a third of body wastes can be lost through the skin in sweat, so a clear skin is a sign of a clean body.

MASSAGE The blood supply bringing nutrients to the skin is enhanced by massage and massage oil keeps the skin supple.

MOISTURIZERS Apply natural products where possible: these protect the skin by replacing water and natural oils that have been lost.

CANCER PREVENTERS Garlic, onions, linseed oil and walnuts are all thought to protect against skin cancer.

Combating external damage

Protect your skin against the ageing effects of the sun with a sunscreen lotion strong enough for your skin type (but see vitamin D, p45–46). Skin tone and elasticity can be reduced by sunlamps.

Smoking dries the skin and smoke contains a number of toxic chemicals that will increase age lines, especially in the vicinity of the mouth and the eyes.

Beauty boosters

The following minerals, vitamins and other supplements will help you to maintain a healthy skin, well-nourished hair and strong nails.

VITAMIN F and other good-quality oils and fats nourish the skin and protect it from dryness.

VITAMIN A AND BETA-CAROTENE act to prevent acne, blemishes and dry skin. They may even help to prevent skin cancer. VITAMIN C reduces the ageing effects of sun, smoke and other chemical pollutants.

VITAMIN E AND SELENIUM minimize the formation of scars and help to reduce the ageing effects of chemical pollutants.

ZINC helps to repair any damage to the skin and to fight any infection that might be present. Zinc is also vital for the health of all the tissues that continue to grow throughout life, such as hair, skin and nails.

SULPHUR the 'beauty mineral', is essential for healthy skin, hair and nails.

THE B-VITAMINS ensure that the new skin cells take up the correct nutrients.

SILICA is found in the skins of fruits and is thought to strengthen human skin. It is also present in HORSETAIL (see p95) and ALFALFA (see p98).

Supplement directory

Many doctors have been taught little about diet and they are, therefore, likely to dismiss the taking of mineral and vitamin supplements as being just a way of producing 'expensive urine'. However, taking mineral and vitamin supplements can be helpful in ensuring that at least the recommended daily intakes are achieved. This is particularly important if you have a small appetite, are trying to lose weight, or when nutritional needs are especially great, for example during convalescence after illness. However, supplements cannot replace a healthy diet.

OFFICIAL RECOMMENDATIONS

For many years government bodies have been trying to estimate what our nutritional needs are. In the United Kingdom, recommendations for the amounts of food energy and other nutrients needed by children and adults each day have existed for over thirty years, and are now known as Reference Nutrient Intakes (RNIs). In the United States, the Food and Nutrition Board first published the similar Recommended Daily Allowances (RDAs) in 1943. In both countries, these recommendations have been revised from time to time in the light of scientific advances. The current recommendations, which are quoted in this chapter, are considered to be sufficient to meet the known nutritional needs of 'practically all healthy persons'.

No formal recommendations have been made for some of the vitamins and minerals described in this book, either because the official bodies making the recommendations have not felt that sufficient scientific evidence was available to do so, or because deficiency does not appear to occur. However, in some cases it was felt possible to provide informal guidance; this is also contained in this chapter.

The Canadian Department of Health has set dietary standards since 1938, which are now referred to as Recommended Nutrient Intakes (RNIs). These recommendations (not included in this chapter) differ from the US RDAs mainly because of differences in the interpretation of the same data and in the definitions of the RNIs and RDAs. However, in an effort to harmonize North American dietary standards, Health Canada is co-sponsoring a review being conducted by the Food and Nutrition Board of the US National Academy of Sciences. This review aims to produce a series of Dietary Reference Intakes (DRIs) which are eventually intended to replace the current US and Canadian values. Reports on calcium, phosphorus, magnesium, vitamin D and fluoride, and thiamine, riboflavin, niacin, vitamins B6 and B12, folate, pantothenic acid, biotin and choline are already available from the US National Academy Press Reading Room (www.nap.edu/reading room).

USING THIS CHAPTER

The RNIs/RDAs are obviously lower for small children, but if you study the tables you will also see they recognize that during adolescence nutritional needs can be greater than they are for adults. The amounts needed by males and females also differ slightly, partly because women usually weigh less than men. Women also require extra vitamins and minerals during pregnancy and when breast feeding.

When using these tables it is important to read the relevant sections in chapters 1 and 2 for the explanation of the notes and cautions. The amounts of vitamins and minerals that you need are very small, and in a few cases too much can be toxic. The figures are given in milligrams (mg) and micrograms (mcg).

SUFFICIENT IS NOT OPTIMAL

The RNI/RDA recommendations were originally designed to be the minimum requirement for the avoidance of deficiency diseases. Although these figures are now somewhat higher than this, many nutritionists believe that these recommendations are still not high enough to ensure that people continue to live a healthy life into an old age that is as free as possible from chronic disease. Such optimal recommendations may one day be available, but as yet there is no way to calculate them with sufficient certainty. In any case, people's individual needs are dependent on many different factors and so probably vary more than has previously been realized.

In addition, the RNIs/RDAs make no allowance for illness or for lifestyle. For example, the RNI/RDA for vitamin C for a young man in his twenties is 40mg (UK) or 60mg (U.S.). But it is estimated that smoking one cigarette uses up about 25mg of vitamin C (as well as many of the B-vitamins), so after less than three cigarettes the entire RNI/RDA could be used up without any being available for a smoker's essential needs.

NUTRITIONISTS TAKE SUPPLEMENTS

Most nutritionists practise what they preach by eating the best diet that they can, and this will generally mean that they satisfy the RNI/RDA recommendations for all nutrients. However, many nutritionists also top up their diets with mineral and vitamin supplements because they believe that this extra source is useful, even though watertight scientific support for doing so is not yet available.

In general, minerals and vitamins are safe in doses that far exceed the RNIs/RDAs and manufacturers of supplements take safety into account when they recommend a dose regime. Nevertheless, if you are taking any mineral or vitamin from more than one supplement, you should seek professional advice to ensure that you are not exceeding a safe dose.

A QUICK GUIDE TO METRIC AND IMPERIAL WEIGHTS

g=gram
mg=milligram or one thousandth of a gram
mcg=microgram or one millionth of a gram

1oz=approximately 28g
3½oz=approximately 100g

Water-soluble vitamins

AGE	DAILY RNI (UK) & RDA (US)							
	VITAMIN B1		VITAMIN B2		VITAMIN B3		VITAMIN B6	
	UK	US	UK	US	UK	US	UK	US
	mg	mg	mg	mg	mg	mg NE*	mg	mg
CHILDREN								
0–3 mo.	0.2	0.3	0.4	0.4	3	5	0.2	0.3
4–6 mo.	0.2	0.3	0.4	0.4	3	5	0.2	0.3
7–9 mo.	0.2	0.4	0.4	0.5	4	6	0.3	0.6
10–12 mo.	0.3	0.4	0.4	0.5	5	6	0.4	0.6
1–3 yrs	0.5	0.7	0.6	0.8	8	9	0.7	1
4–6 yrs	0.7	0.9	0.8	1.1	11	12	0.9	1.1
7–10 yrs	0.7	1	1	1.2	12	13	1	1.4
MALES								
11–14 yrs	0.9	1.3	1.2	1.5	15	17	1.2	1.7
15–18 yrs	1.1	1.5	1.3	1.8	18	20	1.5	2
19–24 yrs	1	1.5	1.3	1.7	17	19	1.4	2
25–50 yrs	1	1.5	1.3	1.7	17	19	1.4	2
51+	0.9	1.2	1.3	1.4	16	15	1.4	2
FEMALES								
11–14 yrs	0.7	1.1	1.1	1.3	12	15	1	1.4
15–18 yrs	0.8	1.1	1.1	1.3	14	15	1.2	1.5
19–24 yrs	0.8	1.1	1.1	1.3	13	15	1.2	1.6
25–50 yrs	0.8	1.1	1.1	1.3	13	15	1.2	1.6
51+	0.8	1	1.1	1.2	12	13	1.2	1.6
PREGNANCY	+0.1**[1]	1.5	+0.3[1]	1.6	#	17	#	2.2
LACTATION								
0–4 mo.	+0.2[1]	-	+0.5[1]	-	+2[1]	-	#	
4+mo.	+0.2[1]	-	+0.5[1]	-	+2[1]	-	#	-
0–6 mo.	-	1.6	-	1.8	-	20	-	2.1
6–12 mo.	-	1.6	-	1.7	-	20	-	2.1
NOTES AND CAUTIONS	• Toxic in high doses		• High doses may cause loss of the other B-vitamins in urine		• Can cause blood pressure to fall • Check with your doctor if you have any medical condition		• Toxic in high doses	

*1NE (Niacin equivalent) is equal to 1 mg Niacin or 60mg dietary tryptophan
**Last 3 months only
[1] To be added to adult requirement
No further addition to adult requirement

Water-soluble vitamins

AGE	DAILY RNI (UK) & RDA (US)					
	FOLIC ACID		VITAMIN B12		VITAMIN C	
	UK	US	UK	US	UK	US
	mcg	mcg	mcg	mcg	mg	mg
CHILDREN						
0–3 mo.	50	25	0.3	0.3	25	30
4–6 mo.	50	25	0.3	0.3	25	30
7–9 mo.	50	35	0.4	0.5	25	35
10–12 mo.	50	35	0.4	0.5	25	35
1–3 yrs	70	50	0.5	0.7	30	40
4–6 yrs	100	75	0.8	1	30	45
7–10 yrs	150	100	1	1.4	30	45
MALES						
11–14 yrs	200	150	1.2	2	35	50
15–18 yrs	200	200	1.5	2	40	60
19–24 yrs	200	200	1.5	2	40	60
25–50 yrs	200	200	1.5	2	40	60
51+	200	200	1.5	2	40	60
FEMALES						
11–14 yrs	200	150	1.2	2	35	50
15–18 yrs	200	180	1.5	2	40	60
19–24 yrs	200	180	1.5	2	40	60
25–50 yrs	200	180	1.5	2	40	60
51+	200	180	1.5	2	40	60
PREGNANCY	+100[1]	400	#	2.2	+10*[1]	70
LACTATION						
0–4 mo.	+60[1]	-	+0.5[1]	-	+30[1]	-
4+mo.	+60[1]	-	+0.5[1]	-	+30[1]	-
0–6 mo.	-	280	-	2.6	-	95
6–12 mo.	-	260	-	2.6	-	90
NOTES AND CAUTIONS	• Toxic in high doses • Check with your doctor if you take medication for epilepsy, or are at risk of pernicious anaemia				• Reduce dose if symptoms occur • Check with your doctor if you, or a relative, have had kidney stones	

* Last three months
\# No further addition to adult requirement
[1] To be added to adult requirement

Fat-soluble vitamins

AGE	DAILY RNI (UK) & RDA (US)							
	VITAMIN A		VITAMIN D		VITAMIN E		VITAMIN K	
	UK	US	UK	US	UK	US	UK	US
	mcg	mcgRE[1]	mcg	mcg	mg	mg	mcg	mcg
CHILDREN								
0–3 mo.	350	375	8.5	7.5	-	3	-[4]	5
4–6 mo.	350	375	8.5	7.5	-	3	-[4]	5
7–9 mo.	350	375	7	10	-	4	-[4]	10
10–12 mo.	350	375	7	10	-	4	-[4]	10
1–3 yrs	400	400	7	10	-	6	-[4]	15
4–6 yrs	400	500	-	10	-	7	-[4]	20
7–10 yrs	500	700	-	10	-	7	-[4]	30
MALES								
11–14 yrs	600	1,000	-	10	(over 4)[3]	10	-[4]	45
15–18 yrs	700	1,000	-	10	(over 4)[3]	10	-[4]	65
19–24 yrs	700	1,000	-	10	(over 4)[3]	10	-[4]	70
25–50 yrs	700	1,000	-	5	(over 4)[3]	10	-[4]	80
51–64	700	1,000	-	5	(over 4)[3]	10	-[4]	80
over 65	700	1,000	10	5	(over 4)[3]	10	-[4]	80
FEMALES								
11–14 yrs	600	800	-	10	(over 3)[3]	8	-[4]	45
15–18 yrs	600	800	-	10	(over 3)[3]	8	-[4]	55
19–24 yrs	600	800	-	10	(over 3)[3]	8	-[4]	60
25–50 yrs	600	800	-	5	(over 3)[3]	8	-[4]	65
50–64	600	800	-	5	(over 3)[3]	8	-[4]	65
over 65	600	800	10	5	(over 3)[3]	8	-[4]	65
PREGNANCY	+100[2]	800	10	10	(over 3)[3]	10	-[4]	65
LACTATION								
0–4 mo.	+350[2]	-	10	-	-	-	-[4]	-
4+mo.	+350[2]	-	10	-	-	-	-[4]	-
0–6 mo.	-	1,300	-	10	-	12	-[4]	65
6–12 mo.	-	1,200	-	10	-	11	-[4]	65
NOTES AND CAUTIONS	• Supplements taken as retinol can be toxic: do not exceed RNI/RDA • Avoid retinol during pregnancy (beta-carotene is safe)		• Supplements can be toxic: do not exceed RNI/RDA • Check with your doctor if you have sarcoidosis		• Check with your doctor if you have high blood pressure or take anti-coagulant medicine		• Synthetic vitamin K (Menadione) can be toxic: do not exceed RDA • Consult your doctor if you take anti-coagulant medicine	

[1] mcgRE = Retinol equivalents. 1 retinol equivalent = 6mcg beta-carotene
[2] To be added to adult requirement
[3] Safe intake (No RNI available)
[4] Safe intake for adults is 1mcg per kg of body weight. For infants, safe intake is 10 mcg per day (No RNI available)

Minerals

AGE	DAILY RNI (UK) & RDA (US)							
	CALCIUM		MAGNESIUM		PHOSPHORUS		IRON	
	UK	US	UK	US	UK	US	UK	US
	mg	mg	mg	mg	mg	mg	mg	mg
CHILDREN								
0–3 mo.	525	400	55	40	400	300	1.7	6
4–6 mo.	525	400	60	40	400	300	4.3	6
7–9 mo.	525	600	75	60	400	500	7.8	10
10–12 mo.	525	600	80	60	400	500	7.8	10
1–3 yrs	350	800	85	80	270	800	6.9	10
4–6 yrs	450	800	120	120	350	800	6.1	10
7–10 yrs	550	800	200	170	450	800	8.7	10
MALES								
11–14 yrs	1,000	1,200	280	270	775	1,200	11.3	12
15–18 yrs	1,000	1,200	300	400	775	1,200	11.3	12
19–24 yrs	700	1,200	300	350	550	1,200	8.7	10
25–50 yrs	700	800	300	350	550	800	8.7	10
51+	700	800	300	350	550	800	8.7	10
FEMALES								
11–14 yrs	800	1,200	280	280	625	1,200	14.8[2]	15
15–18 yrs	800	1,200	300	300	625	1,200	14.8[2]	15
19–24 yrs	700	1,200	270	280	550	1,200	14.8[2]	15
25–50 yrs	700	800	270	280	550	800	14.8[2]	15
51+	700	800	270	280	550	800	8.7	10
PREGNANCY	#	1,200	#	320	#	1,200	#	30
LACTATION								
0–4 mo.	+550[1]	-	+50[1]	-	+440[1]	-	#	-
4+mo.	+550[1]	-	+50[1]	-	+440[1]	-	#	-
0–6 mo.	-	1,200	-	355	-	1,200	-	15
6–12 mo.	-	1,200	-	340	-	1,200	-	15
NOTES AND CAUTIONS	• Avoid magnesium deficiency • Avoid taking long term without good medical reason		• Avoid low calcium levels if magnesium is injected		• Ensure adequate magnesium and calcium intake		• Men and post-menopausal women should take extra iron with caution	

No further addition to adult requirement
1 To be added to adult requirement
2 Insufficient for women with high menstrual losses

Minerals

AGE	DAILY RNI (UK)			AGE	DAILY RDA (US)		
	SODIUM	POTASSIUM	CHLORIDE		SODIUM	POTASSIUM	CHLORIDE
	UK	UK	UK		US[*2]	US[*3]	US[*2]
	mg	mg	mg		mg	mg	mg
CHILDREN							
0–3 mo	210	800	320	0–5 mo	120	500	180
4–6 mo	280	850	400	6–11 mo	200	700	300
7–9 mo	320	700	500	1 yr	225	1,000	350
10–12 mo	350	700	500	2–5 yrs	300	1,400	500
1–3 yrs	500	800	800	6–9 yrs	400	1,600	600
4–6 yrs	700	1,100	1,100				
7–10 yrs	1,200	2,000	1,800				
MALES							
11–14 yrs	1,600	3,100	2,500	10–18 yrs	500	2,000	750
15–18 yrs	1,600	3,500	2,500	18+	500	2,000	750
19–24 yrs	1,600	3,500	2,500				
25–50 yrs	1,600	3,500	2,500				
51+	1,600	3,500	2,500				
FEMALES							
11–14 yrs	1,600	3,100	2,500	10–18 yrs	500	2,000	750
15–18 yrs	1,600	3,500	2,500	18+	500	2,000	750
19–24 yrs	1,600	3,500	2,500				
25–50 yrs	1,600	3,500	2,500				
51+	1,600	3,500	2,500				
PREGNANCY	#	#	#	**PREGNANCY**	+69[1]	#	-
LACTATION				**LACTATION**	+135[1]	#	-
0–4 mo.	#	#	#				
4+mo.	#	#	#				
				0–6 mo.	-	-	-
				6–12 mo.	-	-	-
NOTES AND CAUTIONS							

No further addition to adult requirement
* Estimated minimum requirements for healthy persons
[1] To be added to adult requirement
[2] No allowance has been made for prolonged losses from sweating
[3] Desirable potassium intake may be much higher e.g. around 3,500mg for adults

AGE	DAILY RNI (UK) & RDA (US)							
	ZINC		SELENIUM		COPPER		IODINE	
	UK	US	UK	US	UK	US [2]	UK	US
	mg	mg	mcg	mcg	mg	mg	mcg	mcg
CHILDREN								
0–3 mo.	4	5	10	10	0.2	0.4–0.6	50	40
4–6 mo.	4	5	13	10	0.3	0.4–0.6	60	40
7–9 mo.	5	5	10	15	0.3	0.6–0.7	60	50
10–12 mo.	5	5	10	15	0.3	0.6–0.7	60	50
1–3 yrs	5	10	15	20	0.4	0.7–1	70	70
4–6 yrs	6.5	10	20	20	0.6	1–1.5	100	90
7–10 yrs	7	10	30	30	0.7	1–2	110	120
MALES								
11–14 yrs	9	15	45	40	0.8	1.5–2.5	130	150
15–18 yrs	9.5	15	70	50	1	1.5–2.5	140	150
19–24 yrs	9.5	15	75	70	1.2	1.5–3	140	150
25–50 yrs	9.5	15	75	70	1.2	1.5–3	140	150
51+	9.5	15	75	70	1.2	1.5–3	140	150
FEMALES								
11–14 yrs	9	12	45	45	0.8	1.5–2.5	130	150
15–18 yrs	7	12	60	50	1	1.5–2.5	140	150
19–24 yrs	7	12	60	55	1.2	1.5–3	140	150
25–50 yrs	7	12	60	55	1.2	1.5–3	140	150
51+	7	12	60	55	1.2	1.5–3	140	150
PREGNANCY	#	15	#	65	#	1.5–3	#	175
LACTATION								
0–4 mo.	+6 [1]	-	+15 [1]	-	+0.3 [1]	-	#	-
4+mo.	+2.5 [1]	-	+15 [1]	-	+0.3 [1]	-	#	-
0–6 mo.	-	19	-	75	-	1.5–3	-	200
6–12 mo.	-	16	-	75	-	1.5–3	-	200
NOTES AND CAUTIONS	• Toxic in high doses		• Do not exceed RNI/RDA		• Toxic in high doses			

No further addition to adult requirement
1 To be added to adult requirement
2 Safe and adequate range of dietary intake, but this range should not be exceeded on a long-term basis

Recommended daily intakes for vitamins and minerals that have been estimated to be safe and adequate where no formal RNI (UK) or RDA (US) has been established.

Vitamins

CHOLINE

UK

No recommendation made as it can be synthesized in the body.

US

The average intake from the diet is 400–900mg per day, and is regarded as safe and adequate.

VITAMIN B5

UK

There is no evidence of deficiency in the UK, where the average intake of adults is 3–7mg per day. For infants 1.7mg per day is safe.

US

Age	mg per day
0–6 months	2
6–12 months	3
1–3 years	3
4–6 years	3–4
7–10 years	4–5
11+ years	4–7
Adults	4–7

INOSITAL

PABA (para-aminobenzoic acid)

VITAMIN B13

VITAMIN B15

VITAMIN B17

VITAMIN T

VITAMIN U

UK and US: No recommendations have been made. None is regarded as essential.

VITAMIN P

UK and US: No recommendations have been made.

BIOTIN

UK

10–200mcg per day is safe and adequate for adults.

US

Age	mcg per day
0–6 months	10
6–12 months	15
1–3 years	20
4–6 years	25
7–10 years	30
11+ years	30–100
Adults	30–100

VITAMIN F

UK

The Panel on dietary reference values recommends that linoleic acid should provide at least 1 per cent of total energy and alpha linolenic acid at least 0.2 per cent of total energy.

US

No recommendations have yet been made.

Minerals

BORON

UK and US: No recommendations have been made. Not regarded as essential.

COBALT

This mineral is part of the vitamin B_{12} molecule, and intake is adequate if vitamin B_{12} is adequate (see table on p133).

CHROMIUM

UK

Above 25mcg per day is safe and adequate for adults, and between 0.1–1mcg per kg of body weight per day for children and adolescents.

US

Age	mcg per day
0–6 months	10–40
6–12 months	20–60
1–3 years	20–80
4–6 years	30–120
7–10 years	50–200
11+ years	50–200
Adults	50–200

SULPHUR

UK and US: No recommendations have been made.

MANGANESE

UK

Safe intakes are believed to lie above 1.4mg per day for adults and above 16mcg per kg of body weight per day for children.

US

Age	mg per day
0–6 months	0.3–0.6
6–12 months	0.6–1
1–3 years	1–1.5
4–6 years	1.5–2
7–10 years	2–3
11+ years	2–5
Adults	2–5

MOLYBDENUM

UK

Safe intakes are believed to lie between 50–400mcg per day for adults, and 0.5–1.5mcg per kg of body weight per day for children and adolescents.

US

Age	mcg per day
0–6 months	15–30
6–12 months	20–40
1–3 years	25–50
4–6 years	30–75
7–10 years	50–150
11+ years	75–250
Adults	75–250

SILICON

UK and US: Human requirements are not known and estimates of average intake vary widely.

Glossary

AMINO ACIDS chemical compounds that contain nitrogen and are found in food. The body can manufacture a number of amino acids but others have to be obtained in the diet and are known as the 'essential' amino acids.

ANTI-OXIDANTS substances that prevent free radicals causing damage.

ATHEROMA the fatty deposit on the walls of arteries that restricts blood flow and may block the artery entirely.

CARBOHYDRATE a class of nutrient that includes sugars (simple carbohydrates), and starch and dietary fibre (complex carbohydrates).

CORTISONE a hormone secreted by the adrenal gland that controls many of the functions of the body and enables people to adjust to stress.

DYSPEPSIA indigestion.

FAT a class of nutrient that comprises the fats and oils in the diet.

FIBRE cellulose that makes up cell walls of plants. It is not digested in the body. Helps prevent constipation and to control levels of cholesterol.

FREE RADICALS unstable chemical substances that occur in the body as a result of chemical processes. They are more common when the body is exposed to environmental pollution, and can cause damage to cell membranes and to proteins. They are neutralized by anti-oxidants, which include beta-carotene (pro-vitamin A), vitamins C and E, and selenium.

GLUCOSE simple sugar either present in food or made when more complex sugars and starch are digested. The main source of energy in the blood and the cells of the body. Also known as dextrose.

GLYCOGEN a complex carbohydrate.

HAEMORRHOIDS dilated veins in the anus.

HEARTBURN indigestion.

HOMOCYSTEINE an unsafe chemical that occurs naturally as part of the basic processes of the body, and appears to contribute to heart disease. It is normally made harmless in the body when sufficient vitamins, including folic acid and vitamin B6, are present.

HYPERTENSION raised blood pressure.

LISTERIA bacteria that cause an infection that is usually mild, but can injure a baby if the mother is infected during pregnancy.

NEURALGIA pain in the nerves.

NITROSAMINES chemicals formed from compounds containing nitrogen, including chemical fertilizers and certain preservatives. They have been implicated in the formation of cancers.

NUTRIENTS substances in our diets needed for energy, repair and maintenance of the body and, in childhood, growth. Generally classified as macro-nutrients (protein, carbohydrate and fat) or micro-nutrients (vitamins and minerals).

OSTEOPOROSIS a condition in which the bones become thin, as a result of the loss of both minerals and protein.

PELLAGRA a condition caused by lack of vitamin B3, in which the symptoms are skin changes, diarrhoea and dementia.

PERNICIOUS ANAEMIA a form of anaemia caused by lack of vitamin B12, either in the diet or because the body cannot absorb it from food.

POLYMER a substance that is made up from small units that are identical with each other.

PROTEIN a class of nutrient that contains nitrogen, and comprises a group of linked amino acids. In plants and animals, proteins either form parts of the structure or they enable the basic chemical processes to occur. When eaten, proteins in food are broken down to amino acids during digestion and these can then be used by the body to create the specific proteins that it needs.

PSORIASIS a chronic disease of the skin in which dry scales are formed.

SARCOIDOSIS a disease of unknown cause in which certain cells of the immune system collect together in the skin, lungs and other tissues.

SCIATICA pain in one of the sciatic nerves, which lie in the buttocks and down the back of the legs.

STARCH complex carbohydrate made from glucose polymers.

TOXAEMIA OF PREGNANCY a complication of pregnancy in which the blood pressure rises, the body retains fluid and there is protein in the urine.

Bibliography

THE COMPLETE GUIDE TO SPORTS NUTRITION
SECOND EDITION
Anita Bean
A&C Black, London, 1996

THE DICTIONARY OF MINERALS
Leonard Mervyn
Thorsons, Wellingborough, 1985

THE DICTIONARY OF VITAMINS
Leonard Mervyn
Thorsons, Wellingborough, 1984

DIETARY REFERENCE VALUES FOR FOOD ENERGY
AND NUTRIENTS FOR THE UNITED KINGDOM
Report of the panel on dietary reference
values of the committee on medical aspects
of food policy
The Stationery Office, London, 1991

THE DOCTORS' VITAMIN AND MINERAL
ENCYCLOPEDIA
Sheldon Saul Hendler
Leopard Books, London, 1995

ESSENTIAL SUPPLEMENTS FOR WOMEN
Carolyn Reuben and Dr Joan Priestley
Thorsons, London, 1991

FATS THAT HEAL, FATS THAT KILL
Udo Erasmus
Alive Books, Burbaby BC, 1993

THE FOOD MEDICINE BIBLE
Earl Mindell
Souvenir Press, London, 1995

THE FOOD PHARMACY
Jean Carper
Simon and Schuster, London, 1990

THE HERB SOCIETY'S COMPLETE MEDICINAL
HERBAL
Penelope Ody
Dorling Kindersley, London, 1993

NUTRITIONAL ALMANAC THIRD EDITION
Lavon J. Dunne
McGraw-Hill, New York, 1990

NUTRITIONAL BIOCHEMISTRY AND METABOLISM
WITH CLINICAL APPLICATIONS SECOND EDITION
Edited by Maria C. Linder
Appleton and Lange Norwalk, Connecticut, 1991

NUTRITIONAL MEDICINE
Stephen Davies and Alan Stewart
Pan Books, London and Sydney, 1987

RECOMMENDED DAILY ALLOWANCES 10TH EDITION
Subcommittee on the tenth edition of the RDAs
Food and Nutrition Board, Commission of Life
Sciences, National Research Council
National Academy Press, Washington, 1989

STAYING HEALTHY WITH NUTRITION
Elson M. Haas
Celestial Arts, California, 1992

VITAMIN BIBLE
Earl Mindell
Warner Books, New York, 1979

Picture credits

Index